MAKE HIM COME TO YOU BEGGING!

39 Secrets To Letting Go Of Your Limiting Beliefs and Attract A Guy Instead Of Chasing Him

By
Bryan Bruce

MY GIFT TO YOU CLICK THE LINK BELOW

https://nowthis.life/rac/

PLEASE WRITE A REVIEW!

If this book helped you out in anyway, please help
me to help others by writing a review!

<u>CLICK HERE TO LEAVE A REVIEW</u>

Still, if you did not get anything new from this book or you were
not impacted in some way, I would still like to hear what you have
to say. Either way, I will know what am doing right or wrong and to
improve in the future. I wouldn't like to take your money and not
deliver. So please, take just 2 minutes to let me know what you think.

Everyone is searching for help on how to improve their lives for the
better and one thing they do look for are reviews. If this book has a lot
amazing reviews with great comments, they will buy the book and read
it and so the ripples effects of goodness spreads. But if it doesn't have
any great reviews and comments, they don't buy the book and read it.

I know this book can positively impact and help someone
and you can help that person by writing your
thoughts and takeaways from the book.

Additionally, I would like to read your review and hear how
this book has helped you in anyway at shape or form. My plan is to
print every single review and hang them on my home office wall
to read for inspiration and motivation throughout the day.

Your great review helps me personally to stay focused
and be able to validate all the hard work and lots of hours
invested in preparing this book for you.

https://nowthis.life/rac/

Legal Disclaimer

Although the information in this book may be very helpful, it is sold
with the understanding that neither the author nor the publisher is
engaged in presenting specific psychological, emotional, or sexual advice.
Nor is anything in this book intended to be a diagnosis, prescription, rec-

ommendation, or cure for any specific kind of psychological, emotional, or sexual problem. Each individual has unique needs and this book cannot take into account each of these differences.

TABLE OF CONTENTS

INTRODUCTION

Despite what you might have heard, guys aren't just in it for the sex. It's not that sex isn't an important part of a relationship for a man, because it certainly is.

If you go into a relationship just hoping that a guy will see your value, your entire relationship is likely to be focused around the quality and quantity of your sex which isn't the making of a good relationship. Here's the thing,

The same man who sleeps with one woman and never talks to her again will end up begging a second woman to commit to him. If you want to be the woman who he wants for a committed relationship, you need to trigger in him the feeling that he's met **"the one"** he's been looking for.

In this book, I'm going to walk you through what this secret process is that would make a man come back to you begging and also secrets to attract a guy instead of chasing him.

FIRST STEP: YOU

1- KNOW YOU: HOW YOU CAN UNDERSTAND YOURSELF IN RELATION TO DEALING WITH A GUY TO GET HIM INTERESTED IN YOU

The first thing for you is to let go of your limiting beliefs, know yourself and understand yourself well enough to recognise **what you genuinely want** in a man, not **what you think you want.** Look, I have been in situations where I think I know what I want, but on getting that result, I realise that I actually didn't want what I got but I wanted something else.

A lot of argument can certainly be made when most people say that most women don't really know what they want in a man but I dear say that it also applies to any man and happens to all of us from time to time in different aspects of our lives.

So take it from me, it's highly likely that **what you think you want** isn't **what you actually want**. And to know what you really want requires that you completely know and understand yourself, yourself worth and the power and sense of wonder of woman-hood. There is no hard and fast rule for understanding you, but thinking deeply and the following points will help point you in the right direction.

Release shame about your past and the beliefs that keep you stuck and not moving on
- Shame is such an uncomfortable feeling. You think that if you leave it hidden in the shadows, outside of conscious awareness, maybe, just maybe, you can pretend it's not there. But it is. And the truth is, it's dug in deep.

If shame stays where it is, unseen and unexplored, it will continue to affect you. How? It's behind the self-critical voice in your head, many unsatisfying dynamics in relationships, feelings of lack and unworthiness, and choices that keep you from fully living.

Shame is so personal! It's a painful feeling of humiliation that you've done something wrong or that there's something disgraceful or embarrassing about you. It's the secret emotion that can sit in you like a poison.

And the last thing you want to do is bring it out in the open. You think that all that will do is highlight your worst fears about yourself. But here's the possibility for you the light that can begin to untangle shame: If you explore it skillfully, if you navigate shame with wisdom and heart, you find tenderness, compassion, courageous vulnerability, and the relief that comes from no longer hiding from yourself or keeping yourself hidden from others and the world.

You move from feeling oh, so separate and alienated to being more at ease with yourself and your own experience. The boundaries that disconnect you from everyone and everything begin to fall away.

Almost like being born anew, you are open, light, and available to life. You can make the choice to let your pain rule you by keeping it in the shadows. Or you can befriend, explore, and welcome it into the light of conscious awareness.

Believe you are beautiful and valuable irrespective of your flaws and weakness
- Beleiving in your self and knowing your worth of how valuable you are is the key just remember if you believe you are beautiful others would believe in you. Let me give you an instance; diamonds don't know how valuable they are.

Try complimenting them on something else. Reinforcing their confidence in their intelligence, creativity, athleticism, anything else besides their beauty is always taken well. They probably get "you're so beautiful" all the time, maybe they need a change from the normal. Irrespective of your flaws or weakness believe in yourself then others would too.

Accept yourself and judge yourself less

- If you accept yourself for who you are it would save you from unhappiness and dip depression. It would disregard your belief that others are better than you are or comparing yourself to other women. Fortunately, self-acceptance is something we can nurture. Look at it as a skill that you can practice versus an innate trait that you either have or don't.

Forgive yourself for past mistakes and let go of the mistakes

- Have you ever noticed how you can hold on to past mistakes long after they occurred? Some of us hold on to things for years! Forgiveness is a process. It does not happen over night and the process will be different for everyone.

But no matter how long it takes, there's hope. Whatever doesn't kill you, really does make you stronger. But it's not about physical strength. It's about mental toughness, emotional fortitude, and a spiritual awakening that can only be realized through an enormity of pain.

That pathway of pain leads to understanding, growth, maturity, and of course, forgiveness. Here are some steps you can take toward that journey: Become clear on your morals and values as they are right now, realize that your past is past, realize you did the best you could do at that time, Start acting in accordance with your morals and values, Identify your biggest regrets, and most importantly move towards self love.

Minimize the need for approval to feel more confident

- Sometimes it can seem like our happiness depends on other people in today's society. But there are ways to stop seeking approval of others. The key is to begin with addressing your own thought process.

Rather than seeking approval from external influences, try to find true happiness by developing a more stable relationship within yourself. "It's exhausting trying to be everything to everyone. But more to the point, it's unsustainable.

Eventually the psyche just collapses in on itself, like a sinkhole of muck, pressured by the weight of trying to figure out who other people want you to be. To be truly happy, you must honor the truth of you. Feeling confident without anyone else's approval means loving yourself first and knowing your own self-worth.

The approval you really need to find is from yourself and this can only begin once you stop searching for approval in others and take the time to heal yourself. Often even just the awareness of your actions will provide you with a great deal of healing.

Be sure to take the time to explore your feelings and learn why and where it's coming from. Once you do that then you'll most likely find that you no longer need approval from others for that particular feeling.

Let go of the comparisons that keep you feeling inferior

- We live in a competitive society, which often means that we end up comparing ourselves to others. Am I prettier than she is, Comparing yourself to others can easily become a habit; and an incredibly destructive one at that.

Some of the reasons why you should stop comparing yourself to others:Comparing yourself to others often leads to self-doubt, Constantly comparing yourself to others can fuel mean-spirited competitiveness versus collaboration.

Comparing yourself to others makes your self-worth dependent on the achievements of others. If they're doing poorly compared to you, you feel good. If they're doing better than you are, you feel bad. Do you really think it's a good idea to make how you feel about yourself depend on how other people are doing? Comparing yourself to others sucks the joy out of life. So stop today and live a joyful life.

Feel complete so that you no longer look to others to fill a void within yourself
- When you lose something or someone, all of the wounds, emptiness, pain and hurt are exposed. As much as it hurts, the void should not be feared. The void is where miracles, strength and change are born.

The truth is that anytime you try to distract yourself from feeling what you're feeling, you're avoiding the fact that you're not whole. Something is missing, damaged or broken, and until you face it, no person or thing will ever make you feel complete.

When you take the time to really feel and experience the uncomfortable space that is the void, you begin to see things clearly. And when you can see things clearly, you can begin to heal and feel complete.

Find the courage to share your authentic self for deeper connections with others
- Your role in life don't make you who we are. We tend

to base our idea of who we are on everyday roles such as parents and spouse or even what we do in our jobs or what qualifications we have. We even go to the extent of changing our who we are in different social situations & acting out of character because we think we have to.

Realize that by acting in this way you are not being you at your deepest level. When you begin to find the courage to share your authentic self you will begin to experience the benefits of a happier life.

Benefits of becoming your authentic self Include:Being happier, Feeling of fulfilment, Decision making becomes easier, Awareness increases, Truthful to self & others, Doing things on your own terms, Doing what you really want, Doing what you love, Satisfying your needs, A sense of purpose, Helping you prioritize how you live,Being in alignment with your goals & dreams.

Learn to take care of yourself instead of putting everyone else's needs first

- *"Self-care is never a selfish act it is simply good stewardship of the only gift I have, the gift I was put on earth to offer to others"* quoted by Parker Palmer.

Remember the old cliché? "Take care of yourself first or you will have nothing left to give others." Or, " we can't give what we don't have." But what is self-care really? Why is it so difficult and why do we feel guilty about doing it?

We were all given this special house to live in our own body, mind and soul. For you; it is your responsibility to take good care of it and treat it with ultimate respect. It carries within your special gifts and talents that are uniquely yours.

Self-care is about seeking and nurturing internal validation. As you learn better self-care, you become a better person in general. When you are in touch with your own feelings, you can then reach out more effectively to others and show love and empathy to them also. If you are filling your own emotional tanks with self-respect and loving care.

Believe that you're valuable so you can start creating a life you love

- *"You are always a valuable, worthwhile human being – not because anybody says so, not because you're successful, not because you make a lot of money – but because you decide to believe it and for no other reason."* – **Wayne Dyer, American self-help author and motivational speaker (1940-2015).**

Just because others say you're no good, can't do anything right, are worthless and without value doesn't make it so.

By the same token, what others say about your successes, whether to your face or to someone else, while it's comforting to hear and learn about, also doesn't reflect on your own innate value and self-worth. What does is how you regard yourself.

Each human being has value and worth. It's up to each of us to find those qualities within us and maximize our potential. Self-worth and value are like seeds that require certain conditions in order to grow and thrive.

Without proper care, seeds wither and die, although they may lay dormant for some time waiting for the right conditions to appear again. In the same manner your self-worth and value wait to be cultivated, nurtured, acknowledged and embraced.

It's also worth remembering that no one else can do this for you. You can bask in praise others give you and this is an indication that you're doing something good and right – but words others say don't change who you are and what you're capable of. Only you can do that.

2- THE TRAITS OF A DESIRABLE WOMAN

Not rushing into having sex

- Cool women enjoy sex, but prefer to wait if they are looking for serious commitment. Far from being constrained by "The Rules," they understand that when introduced too soon, sex comes at a heavy price. "Sex releases Oxytocin — the body's love drug.

Many female have sex early and the release of chemicals has them mistaking a virtual stranger for their 'perfect match.' This illusion typically ends in devastation. Desirable women see dating as an opportunity to evaluate different suitors, which necessitates a certain detachment and level-headedness.

By putting sex on the backburner, these women can also distinguish between men looking for a relationship versus those just looking for a good time. Desirable women are in no rush to move quickly, and aren't pressured by anyone's impatience.

Passionate about life

- Desirable women do not cling to or suffocate their partners. They understand that men enhance their lives, but are not their lives. Whereas many women mistakenly merge their lives with their partner's in hopes of greater closeness (this should not become you), desirable women understand that independence actually fuels desire.

Desirable women don't waste time gossiping or worrying about the latest carb-free diet. They are busy milking life for all it's worth and rarely lack for a funny story based on their own experience. These women have separate careers, interests, and/or bank accounts.

Be emotionally stable and resilient

- Desirable women are overwhelmingly agreeable and content, reserving their anger for when it's truly necessary. Yeah, that's right. If you want that guy to see you as a really cool and desirable woman, then you need understand that happiness comes from within.

You can create stability by tending to your emotional needs from a variety of sources, thereby lessening the pressure on your partner. You need to spend time with your girlfriends. Take classes that fuel your passions.

You should exercise regularly to burn off stress. Cool women inherently understand that a balanced life equals a happier relationship and so should you.

know your boundaries, and don't be afraid to communicate them

- Desirable women aren't afraid to speak up, even if it ruffles a few feathers. Cool women are not difficult or high-maintenance. You should strive at all times to be such and at the same time; do expect a certain standard of treatment and don't be afraid to voice your needs. By making your boundaries known, you would attract partners who are deeply respectful and courteous.
-

They don't put the cart before the horse

- In a world that overwhelmingly pressures women to conform to what to eat, how much to weigh, when to marry and have children; desirable women march to the beat of their own drum.

They are worried less about arriving at a certain destination, and more about their companion for the ride.

"It's incredibly devastating to wake up mid-life and realize that your life choices do not reflect you, but were merely an effort to keep up with the expectations of friends, family and society.

I know lots folks going through divorce who regret not putting more forethought into their choice of partner. As it's the greatest predictor of lifelong happiness, desirable girls take their relationship day by day, evaluating how their partner treats them along the way.

They would rather be with the right partner than any partner ans that should be your take too, because life depends on it. Life is just too short, why waste it living in an unhealthy and loving relationship?

3- BE A HIGH QUALITY WOMAN AND TRAITS OF A HIGH QUALITY WOMAN

I wrote about this in particular in my best selling book How To Become A High Quality Woman. You might find it insightful, so go check it out.

A high quality woman has a driven spirit
- No one likes to date a bum. No one truly enjoys having to babysit an Adult and have to carry them through life, while trying to navigate it for yourself, too. For me and am sure most guys, it is important that a lady has some goals and ambition.

This might be to change the world, this might be to have an amazing career, and this might also mean to raise some amazing children with the best upbringing as possible. Whatever it is, you should know what you want and goe for it.

That is sexy to me, and most Women I talk to find it sexy when a guy has this trait as well. Knowing what you want and going for it is a trait you and every women must adopt.

Confidence
- Confidence is the key, There is nothing more painful than dating a Woman who lacks confidence. No one likes the timid Girl who can't communicate like an Adult, or needs her ego to be massaged every second of the day.

The thing is, we all have insecurities, but a High Quality Woman recognises this and just owns it. A lack of true confidence demonstrates a lack of selfworth. And if you don't like herself, then who will? Confidence defines a woman.

Loving and caring

- One of the trait of a quality woman is being loving and caring.

Having your own opinion and sticking to it

- As a high quality lady, you opinions are not necessarily a reflection of your man's and they shouldn't be. Whether it's politics, sports, movies or sometimes, even perspectives on life you should have own experiences to draw from and form your own opinions that you can vocally state without feeling the need for validation.

Giving room for new experiences

- It's great that you know what you like and what you don't like. But sometimes it doesn't hurt to give new experiences a chance. You should make an effort to at least be a part of the activities that your partner enjoys. If it isn't your scene, you can back out- but definitely give it a chance, especially if it's important to your man.

Decision making and standing on whats right

- If you believe in something, you need stick to your guns but don't throw a tantrum or make a scene. Your values and principles we all know are important to you and you can convey that without throwing a fit.

4- HOW TO LET GO SO HE KNOWS YOU ARE PERFECT FOR HIM

Certain things happen before letting go of a man you love, if you are experiencing these list below then you just have to let go
He typically makes plans with you last minute because you are not currently his highest priority.

- When you two do make plans, he cancels last minute repeatedly. He makes every indication that he likes you but may be afraid to lead you on further from that. So he goes along with plans to meet that he may have even initiated himself, but when things appear to get too serious, he unexpectedly pulls back.

He never really asks you out on a proper date. It generally just always feels like you're hanging out. He doesn't call or text you back for days at a time. In other words, he tends to disappear and is inconsistent with the way he communicates. Trust me the bset thing to do is walk away Trust me.

Walk away now, and don't look back. Don't text him. Don't announce what you're doing. Right now, your relationship is imbalanced, and it's time that you balance the scales once more. Here are several things that may help provide some clarity to your situation. While you are not trying to convince him to be with you, you are aiming to make him realize what he knew all along:

Become less interested
- You are likely the one who shows more interest at the moment: in other words, you seem to value the relationship more than he does. But as you withdraw, you

will be signaling that you are not needy and thus not just willing to take whatever he can give. If you are able to genuinely walk away by demonstrating less interest, you will regain the power to guide the relationship. This is also known as the "Least Interested Principle."

Become scarce

- Spend some time away from each other. If he truly appreciates you, he will miss you in your absence and thus want you more. This is also known as the "Scarcity Principle," where we tend to place greater value on something that is rare or taken away from us.

Introduce competition

- Enlarge your network. Become friendly with others of the opposite sex that you are also attracted to.

You can use the dating app Hinge or mutual friends to arrange a few dates. This will not only help you get your mind off of him, but as he inevitably learns through the grapevine or from your social media presence that he now has competition, a healthy dose of jealousy may be an effective way to help him gain clarity about his feelings for you.

As a warning: be authentic in what photos you choose to post or what hints you choose to drop regarding others with whom you are spending time. You are living your life for you, not for him. You should be genuinely trying to have a great time, not just posing and trying to pretend that you are.

This also helps you further develop the "Scarcity" effect. If you genuinely move on with your life, doing most if not all of the above, and he starts to pursue you with texts, calls, and invites to meet like there's no tomorrow – then you'll know that you'll have a boyfriend who ultimately values you.

Remember; if a guy likes you, he will get in touch with you and try everything he can to see you. It's as simple as that. So, if the above starts to work, and you begin to see a greater balance in the relationship, what next?

Get him to invest

- If he finds a way to ultimately stay in your life, let him do so by having him do things for you. While it may be counterintuitive, people tend to like you more if they are doing favors for you, rather than you doing favors for them; after all, we all tend to appreciate more what we have worked hard to obtain and have invested a lot of time and energy into.

This is called the "Ben Franklin" effect. So stop doing him favors, and start asking for them -- ask him to give you a ride, to help you study, to send you something. The more you have him invest, the more you will mean to him.

Reward

- When he behaves in ways that provide more clarity to your situation, and things become less gray and more black and white, be genuinely grateful and reward him for being good to you. Be good to him back; offering him more attention and affection when he does what you like encourages him to continue that behavior.

Maintaining a healthy environment of mutual gratitude is important. So, now, what if he doesn't reach out after you show less interest and take an initial step back? Then it looks like he was not that into you.

He wasn't serious about having you in his life, so why should you invest time and energy to remain in his? Don't reward nonchalance and aloof behavior with your attention. You deserve to be treated with the utmost affection, and it is up to us women to set the bar higher for ourselves in terms of what we are willing to tolerate.

After all, by closing the door on those who are mistreating us or abandoning us at their convenience, we make room for meaningful connections that could lead to unexpected romances and even better friendships. So say goodbye to the grey area, move on, and have fun. Life is short, after all! Spend it with the ones you love and who love you.

SECOND STEP: HIM

1- HOW TO UNDERSTAND A MANS THINKING PATTERN

We know that men are vastly different than women, but did you know that there are ways we men think differently than you ladies? Our minds actually work in a much different pattern than yours do.

Learning about this is helpful because it really sheds light on the differences that you have and why some of your interactions are so perplexing to guys and vis visa. Knowing the ways men think differently than you can be very helpful to you.

For A Detailed Insight In How WE Guys Think Differently Than You Ladies Be Sure to Find My Book *"What We Guys Really Want"* on Amazon

You cannot pressure a man into commitment
- He's either in or he's not. There's really nothing like pressuring a man into something he's not ready for. In fact, this type of pressure can cause a man to run in the opposite direction.

Most serious relationships start to become exclusive within the first few months of dating; and if you feel like you need to bring up where you are, the likelihood is that he might be in a different place.

On the off-chance that your guy just isn't sure of what he wants or doesn't know that you're supposed to talk about it, it's okay to have "the talk." But just know that nothing you say or do during that conversation is going to bring him closer to knowing that you two should be together. Hopefully he already knows that.

And if he doesn't, you'll just be moving on to someone who deserves to be with you. Men mean what they say and say what they mean, ladies (at least sometimes). Rarely when you ask a girlfriend the infamous question "What does it mean when he...." is the answer something mystical. It means exactly what you think it means.

Men love to be taken care of
- "Taking care" of your guy can include a number of things. It can be a little thing like reminding him about his dentist appointment or surprising him with a home-cooked dinner when he gets off work. It also can mean taking care of his ego.

Your man wants you to appreciate that he hung up the curtains without asking him ten times, so showing him that you're appreciative is important. In understanding men, realize that they truly are sensitive beings.

Often women assume their men don't need to hear that they missed him when he's off on an exotic business trip to far-away lands. That his pecs really do look awesome after that 30-minute trip to the gym, or that you do think he's amazing even though his boss doesn't get it. Men aren't wired like women, of course, but they do have feelings.

Ensuring that you understand this about men can literally catapult you to the top of his list of things he can't live without.

What men want in a relationship, respect is number ONE
- Do you feel like you are taking complete control over a relationship? Guess what, ladies? This is not a turn on. While men love a woman who is strong and assertive, she needs to know when to take the lead and when to follow.

Taking complete control in bed, for example, is definitely a turn on. So if you feel like doing the latter, be my guest. Guys love it when their girl takes the reigns in the bedroom. However, don't let your "control freak" need-to-know-right-now nature leak into your relationship.

Trying to be in charge of everything, and belittling things that your guy does will send him away faster than you can say "I think that shirt looks silly."It's important to remember that when it comes to understanding men, you have to get to the core of what they want from you. Respect is a huge "MUST" for most men.

Compliment his achievements (genuinely) and motivate him to be the best man he can be. Understanding men is easier than you think. But if you're still feeling stuck, you may want to find out exactly why your love life isn't where you want it to be with a D-factor Assessment by downloading **Are You For Keeps Or Not**.

2- HOW TO UNDERSTAND THE MALE EGO

The term "male ego" gets thrown around a lot in popular discourse, often without any clear definition. In order to understand how the male ego shapes men's thoughts and behavior, it's important to draw attention to the ways in which it is socially constructed.

In other words, much of what we consider to be the "male ego" is based on long-held assumptions and stereotypes about masculinity and maleness that have social meaning and have been, for the most part, unconsciously internalized by most men. So all you women out there, I want to help you understand the "male ego" as it's called. Often, it gets a bad rap. But it's part of how men are made, and any woman who understands it, has just unlocked the door to her man's heart. So, here goes …

Understand what the "male ego" is
- Analizing from the work of psychologists and psychotherapists in late nineteenth and early twentieth centuries, the ego can be defined most basically as the self. After all, "ego" means "I" in Latin.

The ego is the part of the mind responsible for acting as the "mediator" between the forces and drives of the superego (our conscience and our ideal selves) and our ids (the part that is responsible for satisfying our basic needs).

The ego operates in reality, and is also responsible for mediating between our own needs and how to satisfy them within our environments.

The ego maintains relations with others, reconciling the drives of the id and the superego with the outside world. Many psychologists posited their own theories of the ego based upon Sigmund Freud's explanation of the ego.

In other words, the male ego is not only a reflection of the individual self, but also of cultural definitions of masculinity and ideas about how men should think and act. Men's identities are thus shaped by social influences. Humans are social beings after all.

Understand that gender roles are socially constructed
- In order to understand the male ego, it is necessary to understand how gender roles develop and function in society. Gender roles shape how people think and behave. Gender roles are sets of beliefs and actions that develop within specific cultural contexts and are associated with a particular biological sex (male or female).

The roles help to differentiate between the sexes, so that men are seen to be one way and women another. By occupying these specific gender roles, some individuals function better within their particular social context while others may struggle.

To understand the male ego, you need to understand how society shapes men's expectations of themselves. This is important because most of us have developed ways of dealing with these social demands.

In many cases, we aren't even aware of how society influences us. For example, most of us don't really know how we came to be sports fans or think that blue, green, and gray are boys' colors while pink and purple are girls' colors.

Learn the basic characteristics of the socially constructed male ego
- The male ego is driven by recognition, attention, and action. We are assumed to be more active beings who do important things (such as political leaders, soldiers,

scientists, etc.) and who are deserving of attention by others.

In this vision of the male ego, we are driven by our physical strength, sex drive, and evolutionary biology as competitors for female attention to be competitive, to strive for greatness and power, and to avoid showing any emotion and weakness.

For example, in most American communities, the male gender role is typically understood and described in active as opposed to passive terms. Men are courageous, strong, competitive, independent, and stable (in contrast, women are passive, emotional, weak, and more socially-oriented).

To give another example, men in many communities in the western world are expected to avoid showing emotion. Remember the old saying "boys don't cry?" Instead, men are supposed to be macho and strong in the face of personal challenges, such as loss, grief, and sadness.

Be aware that not all men feel comfortable performing these standard gender norms
- A lot of us feel conflicted about having to be a certain type of man; even yours truly. For example, what about men who are not attracted to women, even though heterosexuality is still seen as the norm in today's society?

Or what about men who enjoy pedicures and facials, things considered "girly" or feminine? It's important to find out how individual men feel about and respond to these social expectations of how men should be because they will vary in each and every case.

How to deal with the male ego
- Male-female dynamics are quite complicated with social standings, expectations, emotions and ego, all get-

ting in between. Both men and women have emotions as well as ego, contrary to popular belief that women have more emotions and men more ego.

But, it is true that while you should never try to hurt a woman emotionally, you should also not mess around with a man's ego. It is a fact of life that men are more egotistical than their female counterparts.

A bruised male ego will take a long time to heal and will take a heavy toll on any relationship. But, this does not mean that the male ego is something to be despised. In fact, many of the protective instincts of men arise from this same ego.

Consider how social expectations shape men's handling of emotions

- All men and women have emotions, even if they show them in different ways. Men who don't show much emotion still have emotions, but because of social conditioning they have learned not to show their emotions as little as possible or not at all.

This might mean that the man in your life might remain stoic when someone important to him dies. Since anger is an emotion that is more acceptable for men to show, in situations where they might be sad, they will instead get angry.

If your man has a reaction that confuses you, keeping this social conditioning in mind will help you understand his reaction. He has emotions, but he's been taught not to show them, because it's perceived as a sign of weakness.

Learn to recognize emotion suppression

- Men are often taught to suppress their emotions, which is not always the most productive way to deal with emotions nor healthy. Suppressing emotions can create a disconnection between emotions and thoughts. This means that we guys might not even know what we're feeling.

It is important for us to work on expressing emotions because emotion suppression can lead to negative physical and psychological effects. Because of emotion suppression, your man might not be able to discuss how he is feeling.

If he's willing to work on this with you, realize that this will take practice and time. Realize that suppressing emotions is not only a male trait. Women suppress emotions also. Women also need to work on expressing their emotions in productive ways. Just because women are thought to be better at expressing emotions, this doesn't mean this is always the case.

People are not born knowing how to express their emotions in meaningful and efficient ways. It's a skill that needs to be learned for both you and your man.

Challenge outdated stereotypes about men and masculinity

- Unlike that old saying, men are not from Mars and women are not from Venus. Men and women are much more alike than many people would like to admit. In fact, many scientists today prefer to discuss gender differences in terms of a broad continuum of possibilities, as opposed to a strict distinction between two straightforward options.

It's important to avoid making assumptions about men and anticipate their behavior to conform to the gender roles and expressions you'd typically expect. Don't assume he likes sports, for example, or that he likes beer and hates "chick flicks", which are all common stereotypes about men.

Take me for example, I don't really care about soccer.

I can't even give the name of any top soccer player in any team. Most guys get so excited and all worked up about but not me.

Rather, get to know the man in your life on an individual level as opposed to approaching him based upon what you think you know about men in general. After all, he's just a human being just like you and has his own thoughts, feelings, and beliefs.

Empathize

- Try to understand where the particular man in your life is coming from when he does something that shocks or upsets you. Women also often feel pressure to conform to prescriptive roles about how women should behave and be feminine. Rather than write him off, perhaps show some empathy and understanding.

In some cases, men don't even intend to subscribe to the male ego, but it just happens since they've been socially conditioned regarding how to act. For example, if a man interjects in a conversation to say that he thinks professional women's sports aren't worth anyone's time, don't just blame his comments on the male ego.

Try to understand that he lives in a world where women's sports really are NOT valued as highly as those of men. In a lot of ways, this attitude isn't surprising; both men and women have been told by society that professional men's sports matter more than women's.

The problem may not be with this individual man, but with society as a whole and how it talks about men, women, and gender roles. Empathy can be an important step on the route to transformation. Once you empathize with how his behavior has been impacted by social expectations and norms, you can then begin to open the conversation to challenge that process.

For example, perhaps broach the subject of why we don't value female athletes as much as male athletes in major sports. What types of social cues have led us to think women's sports don't matter as much, such as the news coverage, salaries, etc.?

This empathy can also come in the form of checking your own instant reactions to moments when your boyfriend, father, or other male friend or family member doesn't conform to gender stereotypes.

For example, if he mentions that he really likes to go the ballet, your instinct based on conventional gender norms might be to consider that "girly" and not very manly. Instead, check those reactions and remember that you too might be part of the problem in validating the male ego.

Get to know his sense of humor

- Studies have found that both men and women use humor as a way to complicate their identities as men and women, and experiment with the boundaries between them. But what is interesting is also how humor functions for men and women in terms of sustaining their particular gender roles in society.

While some men might prefer making jokes that reinforce traditional gender stereotypes, such as those positioning women as inferior to them, other men might instead challenge those stereotypes by making fun of the way men have traditionally considered themselves superior.

How a man jokes about his sense of masculinity and the conventional stereotypes that apply to men and women in his culture can tell you a lot about his personality and his willingness to conform to these stereotypes, many of which are outdated according to recent scientific research.

If he makes a lot of sexist jokes that denigrate women and portray men as superior, you're going to have a harder time breaking down the male ego. The first step is to have a genuine discussion about the unfunny nature of those jokes and to ask him why he makes them.

The hope is that he will realize that these jokes are not funny and that he only does it because everyone else does it too. Making men aware of their behavior and drawing attention to the things that they do that reflect almost unconscious motives can help them to be more conscious about what they say and do.

Become closer and more intimate

- The closer you become with a man, the more you will be able to separate the man's true self from the social expectations placed upon him. Keep in mind, however, that this might take some time, as most men will not be willing to open up right away.

As with most relationships, forging intimacy takes time, whether it's with a love interest or friend. However, as your relationship progresses and you begin to delve into deeper topics about your interests and views on the world, he may be able to let some of those gender scripts go.

Talk and get to know each other. Share private details about your past, stories that give a sense of who you are, how you grew up, and what sorts of things made you the way you are today. Ask the man to reciprocate; you might be surprised by his honesty and how, over time, the layers of the macho male ego slip away to reveal his true colors.

Maybe he will confess that he cried when watching The Notebook or that he hates all organized sports, things that are not traditionally associated with masculinity. In other words, as he feels more trusting and open with you, he may be more forthright about some of the ways in which he is ambivalent about some aspects of the gender role he is supposed to embody.

This will act as yet another avenue for more intimate communication.

3- HOW TO MAKE HIM OPEN UP TO YOU

Getting a man to open up to you and share his feelings, fears, and concerns is not as hard as you might think. Here's the thing: Most men want to be able to feel so comfortable with you that they can be themselves and share what they think and feel!

Why? For the same reason you want to feel more connected to him. It feels so good to be able to be complete yourself with another person!

The problem for him is that he was raised very differently from you. He has learned to keep his feelings to himself. He is afraid that if he shows you what's on the inside, you're going to think he is "less" of a man.

And if he cares about you, he definitely doesn't want that to happen. So if you want him to open up to you, he has to feel safe taking that risk with you. You have to show him that you accept him, as he is.

When he shares his thoughts and feelings, you don't want to judge or correct them. You can model what you want from him by "being real!" Be your goofy, funny, sad, real self with him so he will get that you're okay with real feelings...yours and his.

The communication breakdown between the sexes can often be summed up like this: You like to talk about your feelings; he doesn't. It's not his fault. "Boys are taught to be less emotionally open than girls, "They are socialized by their peers and parents never to cry and to embrace traditional norms of masculinity, like being aggressive." (Those action-hero figures aren't saving the world by negotiating with the bad guy) But the era of the man bun has ushered in a willingness on the part of guys to be less guarded.

Millennial men are more down for deep conversations with their partner, but there are differences in how men and women communicate that can make it seem like he's hiding his feelings. "We all share the same need for love, but men don't always grasp how to use talking as a way to get that."

For a lot of men, physical contact or even just hanging with you is their way of letting you in. Here, some methods to get his lips moving.

Never pressure him

- If there's one thing that will make a guy slam the door to his feelings shut, it's pressuring him to open up to you. Guys are pretty defiant creatures and they will really hate you if you try to force info out of them.

  While most women love sharing every bit of their lives with their loved ones, guys would rather keep certain things to themselves. If they really don't want to open up to you and you keep pressuring him to do so, it'll never happen and you even risk ruining the relationship with him altogether.

  Getting him to open up has to be his decision and not something that you make happen. Just imagine if he tried forcing you to do something you weren't comfortable with. It would more than likely prevent you from ever doing it in the first place because you didn't like being pressured.

Compliment him always

- This might not seem like it has anything to do with getting a man to open up to you, but it actually does. Men fear rejection more than pretty much anything else. When you prove to him that, yeah, you're still really into him, he's going to feel relieved and feel better about letting his guard down.

If he's more insecure, it's going to take him a lot longer to open up to you because he already doesn't feel that he truly "has" you. Boosting his self-confidence can work wonders in getting him to finally open up to you and your relationship will actually be stronger when he feels that you really do care for him.

The best compliments to give him are the ones that compliment his personality and his morals. Those are far more linked to his true emotions than any physical traits he has.

Stay calm

- Definitely, remember this if you really want him to open up to you. If you're super calm when the two of you are having a deep, real conversation, he's going to get more emotional than usual.

You should be calm whenever you're together, though, because if he sees you randomly blow up at little things that he does, how could he ever expect that you'll not freak out at something he confides in you with?

Not only will staying calm help your relationship be healthier, but he'll feel a lot better about opening up to you if he knows you won't make a huge deal about it.

Speak less, listen more

- If you're the kind of person that always interrupts others in order to put your own two cents in, well, this is going to be pretty hard for you. You really have to listen to your boyfriend and truly focus on what he's saying. Don't just tell him what you think right away.

Sure, you can always give him your opinion and have a conversation about it, but you have to listen first and comment second. By doing this you're showing him that you're willing to take in all of the information that he gives you before forming an opinion about it and this will grant him some relief when it comes to sharing personal stuff with you.

He won't feel as though you're going to take a small piece of it and then not understand the rest.

Ask him how he feels

- Honestly, some guys just suck at communicating their feelings and it has nothing to do with not wanting to open up to you. Most guys don't tell you about a situation and then add, "it made me really sad."

And you might not understand why he's so upset about something unless he shares the details with you. So instead of asking more about the situation he's telling you about, ask him about how that situation made him feel. If your man is particularly terrible at this then ask him if it made him feel specific emotions.

For example, if he played really poorly during a sports game ask him if the loss made him feel mad or if his own playing made him sad. This will give him a general direction and he can fill in the rest. The great thing about this is that he may be opening up to you without even realizing it. You're so sneaky!

Open yourself to him

- This isn't a one-sided game. You can't expect him to share all of his deepest, darkest secrets when he doesn't know a single thing about your personal life or how you feel about anything. You'll only get him to open up to you if you actually show him that you can be vulnerable, too.

You have to prove to him that you're willing to share personal stuff about yourself before you can expect that he'll feel comfortable sharing the same kind of things with you. And don't you dare pretend.

He's going to tell when you're not being sincere and that's just going to stop him from ever telling you how he feels about anything in the future. Do this often and you'll find that he'll be willing to make the relationship fair by giving you some of the information you want, too.

Make sure he knows you are always their for him
- Some guys are plagued by the overwhelming feeling that they need to be "the man." Society has told him that they can't show any emotions and they have to be the strong one in the relationship. So really, it's no wonder that your boyfriend shuts down emotionally.

You have to let him know that you're there for him to lean on. You have to show him that you'll always be there when he needs someone to talk to and someone to rely on. So whenever he's in a bad mood or upset for some reason but won't tell you why just tell him that if he wants to talk you'll be there.

This doesn't pressure him to open up but informs him that you do want to help if he'll let you.

Be understanding
- Make sure he gets that you really do understand his situation and whatever it is that's bothering him. When a guy feels like he's on his own and that nobody else understands what they're going through, he's going to shut down and want to be alone.

This means he'll never open up to you if he doesn't think

you'll get what's going on in his head. He might think that there's no point in telling you because you just can't relate and therefore can't offer him any helpful insight.

If you want him to open up to you then you have to make a point to let him know that you understand. You can even go as far to tell him a similar situation that you were in and how it made you feel. This shows him that you really do get it and he'll feel better about sharing his thoughts with you.

Feel his excitement

- It's pretty rare to see a guy get super emotional, but when he does, it's because he's elated about something that he did. He maybe got a promotion, hit a home run at his baseball game, or won some money on a scratch off, you have to be there to boast with him and talk him up to himself.

His emotions are going to be on high alert when he's psyched about something, and he'll probably share something with you that he otherwise wouldn't. Get excited with him and give him a real reason to tell you what's up. You're proving that you're empathetic and will share his good times (and bad times, too).

Don't nag him

- We're pretty sure every guy on the planet says this is the number one reason he and his girlfriend fight. She nags him to do something and he just doesn't do it. So you should definitely avoid nagging him to share his feelings with you (but don't nag him about anything else).

He's going to think he can never make you happy and that he's not good enough for you. He's never going to want to share his true feelings with you if he knows that you could just nag him about those later down the road.

Find different ways to request him to do things instead of nagging and you'll find that he'll be more willing to open up to you and give you an inside look at what's really going on inside his head.

Be careful when sharing opininons

- No, am not suggesting that you should never have an opinion about something because that would be super lame. But you should always show that even though you have your own feelings and thoughts about something, you totally understand that others feel differently and you are totally open to other points of view.

If you have a negative opinion about something really important to him and make it known that you will never feel differently, he will never share his opinion if it's something you don't like. He'll never feel comfortable enough to do so because he'll be afraid that you'll get angry or judge him.

A great way to do this is to state your opinion and then say something along the lines of, "but I can understand that other people would feel differently." Even though he might not feel differently, he will feel more comfortable about sharing other things with you, too.

Be trustworthy

- This won't just automatically happen — you have to be the one to put in the work to ensure that he does trust you. Otherwise, he'll never want to share anything with you. You would never walk up to a stranger that you obviously don't trust and tell them something deeply personal, right?

Well, guys are no different. Since emotions are such a big deal to men, they're going to want to ensure that they can trust whoever they're sharing them with so they know nobody is going to tell the guys that he's really a big teddy bear who cries at the site of puppy dogs.

Trust is something that is built from being open and honest with someone. So don't lie, don't cheat, and don't give him any reason to think that you're untrustworthy.

Ask him why he is holding back

- The truth is that even if you do everything right, he might still have reservations that make him hold back how he's really feeling. If you've tried just about everything and just can't seem to reach him, just flat out ask him if he's having any reservations about you.

Ask him if there's anything you can be doing to help him feel more like himself around you. Not only will you increase your chances of figuring out how he's feeling, but you'll also let him know that you feel kind of distant because he's not opening up to you.

He might have had some experiences that made him more guarded and you may have to put in some extra work in order to show him you won't treat him the same way.

Choose the right time

- Timing is everything when it comes to getting him to finally open up to you. If he's mad or depressed, he's really not going to talk about his feelings. You have to wait for the right moment before you can expect him to really talk.

The best time? Usually, when he's in a really, really good mood. Even if you ask them about something that could be sad or something you know might make them mad, he will be much more willing to talk about it when they're in a good mood.

That being said, watch how he responds when you ask him during different times and adjust your strategy for the next time. For example, if he gets frustrated with you asking about that stuff when he just gets home from work, try asking before bed or in the morning.

Be patient

- Everything in a relationship takes time. You build trust, get to know each other, become intimate. It all happens at different rates, not all at once. Getting him to open up to you is really no different. Be prepared for it to take a long time and wait for him to be ready to open up to you.

Every guy is different and then all trust at different rates. Some guys will pour their heart out to you on the second date and others may takes months before they're comfortable enough to share those deep personal thoughts.

You should definitely be patient and realize that just because your ex-boyfriend let you in awfully quickly it doesn't mean your new man will do the same. If you sit back and let things run its natural course you'll find that he'll start confiding in you more and more and pretty soon he'll be 100% open.

4- HOW TO CREATE THE KIND OF ATTRACTION THAT DRAWS HIM CLOSER

A man is most drawn to a woman when she is at her best. If you know this, then you also know how being at your worst – when worry and stress take over can push a man further away. A man comes closer when you are happy, confident, secure and loving.

When it comes to love, you can positively impact your dating life and romantic relationship by how you approach things. Depending on your approach, men are being drawn to you or are pulling away from you.

Be real
When dating and in the beginning of a relationship, it's common to put your best foot forward because you want a man to like you. Don't let your best foot turn into a façade where you are only showing certain sides of yourself.

Trying hard to appear a certain way (e.g. perfect) doesn't let a man know the real you. Your connection will only stay on a superficial level and is a sure way to get him to pull away. Instead, be your true self by letting yourself be vulnerable and seen for who you are.

Let your guard down and speak from your heart, even if it feels uncomfortable. The more you do so, the closer you will be with each other.

Be secure in yourself
- When you really like a guy, you may cater to what he wants and unintentionally sacrifice your own desires. Continuing to do this may cause him to take advantage of you, make you his doormat and wear down your self-

esteem.

This sends the message that he is worth more than you and shows how insecure you are. Being secure in your own skin is attractive and intriguing to a high quality man. Do things that are in line with your integrity and don't compromise your core values.

Accept him

- There's nothing wrong with encouraging a man to improve himself as long as he wants to. But, don't take on a man as a fixer upper project hoping he will change. If you keep trying to change him, he won't feel accepted for who he is and will keep withdrawing.

Accept and embrace him for who he is – the good, the not so good and the quirky. (If his not so good is immoral or unethical, you may want to consider leaving.) Focus on his wonderful qualities and you will get more of the same.

Call him out on things that matter

- One beautiful aspect of being together is to help each other become your best selves. If a man is doing something that is questionable (i.e. out of integrity, shifty or shady), don't look the other way and pretend it never happened. Instead, bring it up to him in a caring and non-confrontational way.

For instance, you can say something like, "We're all human and sometimes do things in ways that make us wish we had done them differently. I've done things that I wasn't very comfortable with. How do you feel about the way things were handled? If you could do this again, what might be different?"

Don't sweat the small stuff

- Don't go on and on about the same things and confront

a man about things that don't matter. You will seem like a nag and he will feel like his every move is being scrutinized. He will think that nothing he does is good enough and distance himself even more.

Don't take things personally

- Keep in mind that it's not what a man says; it's what you make it mean. If a man is in a bad mood or has had a hard day, the way he says things may rub you the wrong way. If this happens, don't take it personally and don't make it mean something bad about you. It has more to do with what's going on with him.

Give him space

- Time apart in a relationship is healthy. While it's essential for both people to spend time together, it's just as important to do things separately. Give a man the freedom to spend time alone doing things he loves and getting together with the guys.

When you willingly give him space, your time together will be more precious and bring him closer. Give him space when he is stressed or working through a difficult situation. You can give him space and still be there for him. He will feel less pressure and appreciate figuring things out with no added stress.

Trust him

- Don't be suspicious of every move a man makes just because you have trust issues. Without trust, this shaky foundation can collapse at any moment. If you don't trust a man, you may think of him as guilty until proven innocent.

Take the approach of innocent until proven guilty. Whether your trust issues stem from being cheated on or being exposed to men who aren't trustworthy, it's best to turn inward and work on trusting yourself to make better choices.

Be loyal
- Don't try to make a man jealous deliberately because you want his attention. This might sound counter to my earlier point but there is a difference between taking genuine interest in other guys without flirting. If you are flirting with and kissing other guys, you may get his attention for the time being instead of keeping it for the long run. Be loyal – it's a quality that good men value in a woman.

5- THE ULTIMATE FORMULA
FOR MALE ATTRACTION

The principle of seduction is the show to attract any man whether you want to seduce your man or you want to seduce any man. It really comes down to hitting that "hidden switch" that turns the man on. I'm sorry to say here that this specific switch is different to every man.

Sometimes it is not even related to physical build-up of the men, it can be a word, an image in his head, an expectation. On other times you can trigger it with a simple smile, a lascivious look (the kind of looks that shows strong sexual desire), a seemingly coincidental touch.

The power of scent
- The scent is one of the most powerful subconscious influences that affect our judgments. In a survey 89 % of the men revealed that the scent can enhance the attractiveness of a women. 55 % of those polled men went a little further and admitted that they would get amorous with a women just because of her appealing scent.

Do you believe that? You'd better do! Everybody who has seen or read "Perfume: The Story of a Murderer" would know what I'm taking about. The scent is one of the most powerful subconscious influences that affect our judgments about the other sex. The way you scent is a vital factor of your success in seduction.

You can compare it to pheromones in the animal world. A woman can enhance her natural pheromones by using aromatherapy oils like sandalwood, rose, ylang ylang, jasmine and patchouli.

They are known for their aphrodisiac properties. Shakespeare wrote, that Cleopatra received Marc Anthony on a ship with perfumed sails. The exotic scent made him fall in love with her immediately.

Even that hopelessly that he gave his life for her. Use a perfume that you like but be careful not to overdo it. Use it sparingly and apply it to your body's so called pulse points: wrists, behind your ears, in the bend of your elbow, behind your knees and on the inside of your ankles.

You can also try to spray the perfume in the air in front of you and walk into the mist. Make your perfume a recognizable part of you. Make your scent imprinted in his mind.

Meeting point "the where factor"
- Believe me, the "where" is very crucial to your success. Choosing a Sports-Bar with the Superbowl on may not be crowned with success. A private dinner with the appropriate romantic ambiance on the other hand will give you the best chances.

Choose places where you can minimize distractions (and ideally competition). You must have his complete attention. Besides, the proper surrounding can be very stimulative. Never underestimate the power of candlelight and the adequate soft music.

Don't reveal it all; show a little, but hide a little more
- There is a certain way to dress that drives men crazy. And I certainly don't mean going slutty. This is a turn-off for most men. You need to find a compromise between showing and hiding your womanly qualities. It's the right combination that makes the secret. I like women, who enhance certain body regions without ac-

tually showing anything.

Steer clear of the obvious. It is very important that you actually feel sexy. And don't forget some killer-lingerie and sexy accessories like bracelets and necklaces.

Be super-confident

- Have the confidence of a super-model. Be a woman who knows what she wants and how to get it. Do you know how to do this? But be aware: there is also a thin red line, if you overdo it, you will most likely look arrogant instead of confident.

You don't want that. Nobody likes arrogance. You can start with renewing yourself, get a complete fresh-up: a new haircut, clothes, start loosing weight. Never underestimate what a new haircut can do to you.

Also watch your posture: keep a straight back and your shoulders backwards, expose your chest. Do everything that makes your confidence boost. Men are very impressed by confidence.

Send signs of interest

- Now it's time to spread a little hope that the man have actually a chance on you. Send him little signs of interest from time to time that make him come forward. Pick some fluff of his jacket (even if there is none!).

Face him directly and slightly lean forward every now and then. Show unclenched hands. Play with your hair or caress other objects. Push your fingers through your hair. Wet and bite your lips from time to time.

Here again; do not overdo it! Experienced men can read these signs, the unexperienced, well, they feel that something's going on.

Killing eyes– the French technique
- Start with almost accidentally sidelong glances. You can follow up with a direct look. Now something starts what can be described as playful innocence (someone once said to me that the French girls invented that): The moment he looks back you instantly lower your eyes and put on an embarrassed smile.

You can even emphasize that some moments later by looking again, this time longer and then again lower your eyes. This is flirting without talking (we can learn a lot from the French, when it comes to lovemaking).

Touch him "accidentally"
- When you reach for something, try to accidentally touch his hand. Don't make it too obvious. Also touch him briefly during the conversation to make a point or when he just made an interesting remark about something.

The secret is being playful with casually touches now and then. This creates tension and also a physical connection. And more importantly: it subconsciously communicates that you're not interested in "only being friends".

The power of erotic dancing
- This one is short and simple: learn how to dance in an erotic way and look for an opportunity for him to see. Don't underestimate the power of this. Most women love to express themselves on the dance floor. Why not learning it and doing it the right way? There are courses on this, or just go to a club, watch and learn. This is very powerful.

Anticipation magic
- Now, here's a good one. This is a variation of "play

hard to get", which by the way is a very doubtful thing. If overdone it will harm you more than being of use. Instead, play a little game called "anticipation".

Anticipation, excitement, and tension can be a huge turn-on for a man. Delay the gratification. Make two steps forward, one step back. Create a strong feeling of dissatisfaction in him. A dissatisfaction which can only be resolved by having you.

It must never seem to be easy for him. Make two steps forward, one step back. Contradict Yourself! Use the before mentioned signs of interest, then suddenly show disinterest, ignore him for two minutes. Then start again. Two steps forward, one step back.

The secret ingredient

- Now, there is a final ingredient to a successful seduction of a man: He must not feel seduced. He must think that he seduced you, not the other way around. Give him his victory, let him be the hero. Men like that. It gives them a feeling of security.

These are some other useful tips in short:
Be mysterious and playful, Awake the explorer in him, Let him do most of the talking, Flirt intensively with 90 % body-language and only 10 % with words, Contradict yourself, confuse him, Try to make an all-senses-explosion: looks, taste, music, touch, scent, Take care never to appear too needy, There you have them, the powerful tips on how to attract any man, get his attention and occupy his brain.

6- HOW TO TRIGGER HIS BASIC INSTINCTS

When you are dating a man who seems to be sending mixed signals, or you are just not sure what he is after, you might be experiencing confusion and frustration.

No matter what your relationship goals are, you should not proceed until you know what his basic instincts are, but discovering a man's intentions can be fairly straightforward.

Look at his body language
- when he talks to you. Good eye contact, a body that is squared up to yours and arms that are spread wide and not crossed are all signs that he is interested in you.

Tell him what your intentions are
- Whether you are interested in a no-strings attached relationship, or something that has long term possibilities, let him know and see how he reacts. If you stop hearing from him after telling him what your intentions are, you were not compatible with each other at that time.

Examine what they do, rather than what they say
- Look at how he treats you and how much he values your company. If you are a priority in his life, it can mean that he is interested in further developing your relationship.

Allow him to contact you
- If a man calls regularly to set up dates or to chat, that is a sign that his interest is strong. Men who are strongly interested do not wait to be contacted, but remember to do your fair share of reaching out as well. No one likes to think that they are making all the effort.

Ask him

- When it doubt, be blunt and ask him what he wants out of a relationship with you. Be specific and be aware that you might not like the answer. However, this is likely the quickest way to get a correct answer and it removes guesswork.

7- 5 WAYS YOU SABOTAGE HIS ATTRACTION FOR YOU AND HOW TO STOP IT

Relationships are really quite simple when you understand the core dynamics at play. When you don't, however, you can drive yourself half insane trying to figure it all out.

The beginning of a relationship is often the most confusing time, a time when everything seems precarious and you don't quite know where you stand or where, if anywhere, the relationship is going.

Men and women are different and as such, the way we experience and process relationships is different. Men tend to be much more in the moment, if the relationship is enjoyable in the here and now, they're happy.

If it's unpleasant, they either distance themselves or leave. Women, on the other hand, tend to get stuck in the details, the nuances, the "clues" both real and perceived. In the midst of this quest to figure out what's going on and where he stands, they often lose sight of what's important (the actual relationship, and how it is in the here and now).

No one intentionally seeks to sabotage their relationship (at least, not if you really like the guy). Conversely, women usually go in with the best intentions and can be blindsided should the relationship crumble before it really gets going.

1- Jumping the gun
- This scenario might sound familiar to you. You meet a guy and instantly hit it off. You go out a few times and realize that he basically has every quality you want in a man. You don't want to do it … but you can't help but think how perfect it would be if it worked out and you

ended up together.

You think about all the crazy coincidences that lead to you meeting him (if there weren't any, you'll find some to make this a great "how we met" story!), and feel certain that this union was written in the stars. You're not even official with him yet, but you could never conceive of dating another guy that would almost be like having an affair! You're sure this guy is the one, you're positive of it.

You have an amazing time together, you talk for hours, things are great except you're on two completely different pages! You think about all the crazy coincidences that lead to you meeting him (if there weren't any, you'll find some to make this a great "how we met" story!), and feel certain that this union was written in the stars.

You're not even official with him yet, but you could never conceive of dating another guy…that would almost be like having an affair! You're sure this guy is the one, you're positive of it. You have an amazing time together, you talk for hours, things are great except you're on two completely different pages!

What's the harm, you might wonder, it's not like he knows you've already picked out the china pattern for the wedding reception. Oh but he does. They always do. Men are not the boneheads sitcoms would have you believe. They are very much in tune with the vibe and energy a woman gives off.

And when a man feels that pressure, even on the slightest level, he will back off. When this happens, you will, of course, start to panic and will cling even tighter, thinking you'd be a fool to let the love of your life slip away!

The more you push, the more he pulls away until there's nothing left but the memory of him and the pain of thinking what might have been.

2- Overanalyzing

- You meet a great guy and you can't help but feel a little worried that your feelings won't be reciprocated. In an attempt to protect yourself, you look at the clues and try to figure out what everything means.

If something seems like a bad sign, you focus on solving it, stat! You pick apart his texts and e-mails, you debate endlessly over what to respond and whether an emoticon would seem cheesy or cute, you spend hours talking to your friends about why he's taking so long to text back and what it means and what he might be up to.

You replay every moment of every interaction with him, keeping a tally of the signs he likes you and signs he doesn't. It's exhausting. I'm exhausted just thinking about it! The truth is, 90% of relationship problems wouldn't exist if women would stop obsessing and analyzing and just go with it.

The more time you spend thinking and talking about him, the more you're investing in him and the more hurt you'll be if the relationship ends. Guys like their relationships and their lives to be simple and drama-free.

The most attractive woman to a guy is one who goes with the flow and can be present in the relationship without putting so much pressure on it. If you are playing "emotional detective," you'll be too busy worrying about the relationship to actually enjoy it!

The best attitude to have is one where you feel happy with your guy, but would be OK without him. Don't waste your time trying to figure out if he likes you and what he meant when he said XYZ, instead be confident and trust that he does like you because why wouldn't he? And if for whatever reason he doesn't, who cares?! You'll find someone else who does.

3- Being official before you're actually official

- Okay, now this is by far the biggest relationship-ruining mistake. Girl meets boy, girl really, really likes boy, girl cuts off all other potential suitors and focuses exclusively on boy even though they never decided to be exclusive.

How this usually turns out is boy tells girl "I like our relationship as it is and don't want to label it" and girl is devastated but stays in the relationship anyway, hoping he'll change his mind. Sound familiar?

I know I for one have been down that road and it sucks! Look, I know it's tough to keep your options open when you find a guy who shines so much brighter than the rest, but you cannot act like his girlfriend until you are his girlfriend.

Why? Because no guy is going to willingly deepen a level of commitment unless he has to. It's not that guys are anti-monogamy, or don't want to commit, it just isn't a man's natural inclination to want to be tied down.

A man will only commit himself to a woman if he is inspired to and if it has a benefit to him. If he is getting all the benefits of having a girlfriend without the obligations that come with being in a relationship, then why in the world would he change that situation?

If you don't necessarily want to date multiple guys at a time that's fine, just do not act like his girlfriend until you are. Don't take down your online dating profiles or prioritize him over everything else in your life or invest in him any further until he reciprocates.

4- Dropping your life for him

- This is another common relationship trap. You start seeing a guy, you spend more and more time together, and suddenly, he is just about the only thing you have going on in your life. You ditch your friends for him, don't go to the gym as often, don't go to book club.

The reason this guy was drawn to you in the first place is because you had a well-rounded, fulfilling life that you enjoyed. You can't expect to abandon that and have him feel the same level of attraction and intrigue towards you. As I've previously discussed, men have an innate fear of being tied down.

It doesn't mean men are anti-relationships or commitment-phobes, it's just the nature of a man to want to go out and spread his seed, if you will. When you abandon all the other areas of your life, it forces him to fill in the empty space and be the sole source of your happiness and fulfillment.

That is way too much pressure for anyone to deal with! Also, if you give up all these things for him and come to expect him to do the same for you, he will begin to resent you for reigning in on his freedom.

The point is, don't stop being who you were before the relationship once you're in a relationship. Keep your life balanced, fun, and fulfilling with many sources of happiness.

5- Not seeing the relationship for what it is

- When it comes to relationships, the devil is in the delusions. Women have such an amazing ability to see exactly what they want to see. A guy might say he doesn't want a relationship with you but you stick around, knowing with certainty that he'll change his mind.

You convince yourself that he doesn't really mean it, he's just saying it. You are positive that he cares about you because he took you to a fancy restaurant, he said he missed you, he told you about his hopes and dreams... any nice thing he said or did from the time you met is tallied up and used as proof that he really cares.

And all the stuff he did that indicates he isn't serious? Well, we can just ignore those and take a glass is half full sort of approach! Before entering into a relationship, you must get clear on exactly what it is you want.

If you don't, then it's far too easy to get caught up in something you don't want. I get so many questions from women who are upset or angry at their guy for reasons that are completely invalid.

For instance, he told her he doesn't want to be exclusive, she continues seeing him anyway, and then she gets mad at him when she catches him texting another girl. So basically, she's mad at him for not acting like he's in a real relationship even though they are not in a real relationship.

To help you get clarity, try making a list of the three traits you absolutely need in a partner, and three deal breakers. Next, get clear on what kind of relationship it is you want. It's okay to admit that you want to get married, or be in a committed relationship.

I know in this day and age it's considered passé for a woman to admit to such things, and instead being independent and strong and not needing a man is all the rage, but if that's what you want, give yourself permission to want it. The only way to ever get what you want is to know what it is.

Why women sabotage healthy relationship with men

While a woman basketball star can say to herself and others that she wants to be in a relationship with a man who is healthy and functional, it doesn't mean that she will be attracted to a man who is like this.

This can relate to woman who can't seem to attract a guy that is healthy and for women who do attract them and yet sabotage the relationship shortly after. And just because one can feel attracted to someone, it doesn't mean that this attraction is a good sign.

And as this challenge shows, one can be attracted to someone that is unhealthy and even dangerous. What they are attracted to doesn't enhance their wellbeing, it compromises it.

The Ideal
- Their ideal man could be one who is: loving, supportive, reliable, confident, trustworthy, respectful, kind, generous, funny, honest and strong for instance. Someone who not only listens to what they have to say, but who cares about what they do say.

For some women the requirements will vary, but the ideal is unlikely to be man that is abusive in any way. They will be there during the good times and where everything is going well and when there are bad times and challenges need to be dealt with.

Reality
- However, although this can be the idea that they have in their mind and what they tell their close friends that they want for example, there is a disconnection. The kind of man they are attracted to is nothing like what they say they want.

In fact, he could be the complete opposite. And then there are going to be women who do find their ideal man, but he may well be lost as soon as he is found. How long this relationship will last will depend on different factors.

There is of course the possibility that a woman could gradually adapt to the healthy relationship. One thing it can depend on is how aware they are.

The Dysfunctional Man
- As this is a man that is nothing like what they say they want, the traits are going to either be the opposite of what they wanted or as what could be described as pseudo versions. So instead of confidence will be arrogance or it will be physical strength in the place of emotional strength.

And this is man that could be: dishonest, unsupportive, unreliable, disrespectful and disingenuous. There could also be some kind of emotional, physical or verbal abuse that regularly takes place.

It Doesn't Feel Right
- It is clear to see that there is a massive difference between these two men. And this is why some women will either not attract a man who is emotionally healthy or end up clash royale hack sabotaging a relationship with a man that is.

Even though there is the conscious desire to be with a healthy man, at a deeper level, they only feel comfortable with men that are dysfunctional. In this situation, the mind and body are not in alignment, they are fighting each other.

Consequences
- So a woman can know what she wants and even

experience it and when she does, a gangstar vegas hack tool online sense of unease will arise. And this can play out in many different ways. The desire to have a man that is reliable can be there and yet when the man is reliable, it doesn't feel right. What would feel right is if he was unreliable.

He could be respectful and treat the woman as his equal and while this is what she consciously wants, it feels wrong. If he was disrespectful, it would feel fine and even normal. Another thing that can create unrest is if the man is peaceful, calm or down to earth for instance.

What basketball stars hack ios the woman feels comfortable with is drama and the highs and the lows; so fighting, arguments and uncertainty. On some level, this kind of man will not be stimulating enough and could be perceived as boring.

What's Going On?

- This can be hard to comprehend for the woman who is experiencing this conflict and for the man who has treated a woman so well and ends up being left. If a woman's body was in sync with her mind, then these problems would not exist.

And the kind of man a woman will be attracted to and feel comfortable with, will typically be the result of what her father was like. So this will be how her father treated her and how he treated the women around her.

Expectations

- During this time, a woman will form expectations of what men are like and what they are not like. And how her father treated her, can then become how all men will treat her. It won't matter if his behaviour was functional or dysfunctional, as the woman will gradually feel comfortable with the behaviour, regardless of how healthy it is.

So if the father was emotionally healthy, it would have created a good model for the woman to internalise. But if this wasn't the case, a woman can end up internalising something that will cause her problems until this model is changed.

This could have been a father that was abusive in some way. Perhaps he didn't have healthy boundaries and ended our going into his daughter's personal space; causing her to feel: overwhelmed smothered, taken advantage of and compromised. Or maybe he was unreliable, always making promises and yet breaking them.

Awareness
- What will need to occur here is for you to feel uncomfortable with men that are abusive and comfortable with men that are healthy; for the body to be working with the mind and not against it.

The early experiences that a woman had with her father would have resulted in certain feelings being created and they could have become trapped in the woman's body. These feelings are causing the conflict and defining the kind of man that they are attracted to in later life.

So as these feelings are released from the body, the kind of men they feel comfortable with will begin to change. This can be done with the assistance of a therapist or healer who will allow them to face their feelings and release them.

THIRD STEP- NOW THE SECRETS TO LETTING GO OF YOUR LIMITING BELIEFS AND ATTRACTING THE ONE

1- Don't Send Mix Feelings

- Having mixed feelings in your relationship often causes confusion and can leave you feeling uncomfortable, exhausted, and stuck. The term "mixed feelings" is having multiple and often competing emotions about your man. Mixed feelings occur when you feel jealous in your relationship thinking all the time if he is cheating on you or maybe he has someone else, this actually causes mixed signal.

In order to deal with mixed feelings towards your man, you need to identify your own feelings, look for a solution, and ask for help when you need it. Not sending mixed feelings in your relationship is one of the key secret in keeping a man.

2- Let Him Be The Man

- When you let a man lead, you can observe what he will do to win you over without your prompts. This is essential to judge his interest level. Does he take three weeks for a second date and more than a week between calls? Or does he ask you for a second date within three days?

Obviously the quicker he gets in touch with you and asks you out, the greater interest he is showing. In this case, texting does NOT count. But, as the woman, if you can't take the wait or think it's unnecessary to let him lead, you might make the mistake of calling and asking when you can see him again. "Are you busy this weekend?" might slip out of your anxious lips.

This is a very bad dating strategy. Now that women and men have achieved greater equality in the work place, women often think its perfectly fine to chase men. They want to be direct and say what is on their minds, ask a guy out, call him if they want to talk. Unfortunately dating has not caught up with work.

Dating is still an archaic mating ritual based in biology. And you can't take the DNA out of dating. What does that mean about the DNA? See a man has hunter instincts coded into his DNA. The hunter wants to win. He enjoys setting his sights on a woman and then doing what it takes to win her over.

He wants dating you to be his idea. Once you are into relationship (after 8 dates approximately) then the chase is mostly over and the dance balances out. But as the woman, if you don't wait, you can lose big time. Men don't like to be chased or pursued. Instinctively, most men (at least men over 40) know this is their job in dating. So when you step in, it's often a turn off.

There is no resistance. No wondering if you like him or not. No striving to win you over. When you call him or ask him out early on, you take all the guess work and mystery out of the situation and a man loses interest.

What makes a man get more interested in you? When he gets invested in winning you over! so when you make yourself too available by initiating contact or asking him out, you ruin the magic and eliminate the mystery. Instead of appearing independent and confident, usually you end up looking aggressive, needy or desperate!

3- Appreciate Him

- If you want to have a long lasting and successful relationship, one of the key aspects you need to keep in mind is to make him feel special in the relationship. Make your man feel loved in the relationship, and he'll feel wanted and desired in the relationship.

And when he feels desired by you, his love for you will grow, and he'll be more eager to please you and win your affection back too. Don't be nice to your man with the sole intention of getting him to reciprocate your gestures and affection back at you.

Do it selflessly because you want to. After all, that's the way true love works. Give something unconditionally because you want to, and if your partner truly loves you back, they'll reciprocate with more love and affection than you gave them! Any day is a good day to appreciate the wonderful man in your life.

When you have a great partner who supports you through all of life's ups and downs, it's important to let him know how much he means to you.

Ways to show you appreciate your man

1. Always start with food:
Everyone knows that the way to a man's heart is with food. It may sound a little old fashioned, but we've never met a man who wasn't happy to have his lady get the stove going and make him his favorite meal! Don't know how to cook? Fake it there are awesome services like Plated and Blue Apron that help you get all the right ingredients and the perfect recipe for a romantic evening so you don't have to.

2. Take him out to events he'll love:
If your guy has a special hobby or loves going out to events, do your research on places to take him and treat him

to a fun date! It'll show him that you pay attention to the things he loves and that you're willing to put in effort to make sure he has a good time.

3. Look him in the eye:

It's one thing to thank your man when he does something thoughtful, but it's another to look at him with love and admiration in your eyes. Slow down. Give him eye contact when you tell him you appreciate him—and give him a big, long, hug when you do. He'll thank you later.

4. Give back when he does kind things:

Remember that time he sent you flowers at work just because? Reciprocate! Your man shouldn't be the only one doing random acts of kindness in your relationship. Return the favor by sending him a chocolate bar at his desk when he least expects it. Hand him a nice cold beer when he gets home. Record the game for him when he can't make it to the TV in time to watch. Anything can work! Just be creative.

5. Give him space:

If life gets a little hectic and your relationship is getting a little tense, you might just need to give your man some space. Men sometimes grow distant when relationships get a little intense.

Rather than suffocate him when you start doubting his feelings, give him time to process his feelings on his own. Your relationship could turn out much healthier and resilient for it.

6. Surprise him with thank you notes:

Showing your appreciation for your man doesn't have to take a lot of time or money that you don't have. Something as simple as a heartfelt note left in his suitcase or in his packed lunch could go a long way.

7. Praise him in front of your friends:

It's one thing to tell your man that you're proud of him in private but it's a whole other story when you do it in public.

The next time you and your friends get together, don't be ashamed to brag about that sweet, thoughtful date your bae took you on last weekend. Your friends might get jealous but your man will hear loud and clear how much him impresses you.

8. Listen to what's on his mind—even if you don't care:

Guys don't talk about their feelings much but when they do, it's important that you hear what he has to say.

Whether it's as major as a huge argument he had with his family or as trivial as a petty spat with a co-worker, give him your undivided attention. Everyone needs to vent even your man.

9. Let him chill with the guys:

Just like you love the occasional ladies night, your man should be able to enjoy the same freedoms without any guilt or restrictions. Let him stay out late and talk to the guys. Sometimes he needs a testosterone fix just as much as you do.

10. Ask him for his advice:

There's no better way to show that you value hearing what someone has to say than to ask them for their opinion.

If you're having a problem with something, whether it's related to work, friends or family, get his perspective on it. He'll feel included in your life and he'll know that you take what he thinks into consideration.

4- Men Need Respect

- The Sole key to keeping any man is RESPECT. A man doesn't just deserve respect, he needs to be respected, it is part of his nature as leader, protector and provider. The need for respect is at the core of his self-esteem, and it affects every area of his life.

Women will have to meet her man's need for admiration and respect by understanding his value and achievements. She needs to remind him of his capabilities and help him to maintain his self-confidence.

The way man was made is to be respected; it is expected of every woman to give man the respect he need. This not take away respect for woman as well, both man and woman need respect of course but man need it much more than woman need.

A Woman'S failure to show this needed respect to her man is one of the many of the reasons why relationships collapse. Respect is the one thing a man needs to feel masculine and commendable.

Men are not safe with anyone who doesn't respect them, either male or female, and they will and should avoid disrespectful people at all cost. Respect keeps your lover safe, gives space for your male children to grow up, and teaches your female children to stand proud.

Love should be submissive to respect, because in the absence of respect, love rots all emotion. Love is just like water, extremely vital to life, but if love is in a wrong place it drowns anything in it.

Respect is what keeps love where it nourishes and grows things, never mind your sexual category or age. No matter how self-assured men may appear on the outside, on the inside they are all secretly harboring massive insecurities about not being worthy enough – not having what it takes to be a 'real man'.

Underneath that confident exterior, your man may be feeling helpless, dumb, ugly, weak, or boring. And he's looking to you to either confirm or deny his fears. A lot of how he feels inside comes from how he sees himself in your eyes.

Did you know that a recent survey showed over 40% of men feel unappreciated by their significant others or families? If he is not feeling respected by you, whose opinion matters to him most, how is he meant to gain the respect of anyone else?

For him to feel loved and worthy as a man, he needs to feel respected by you. And for him to feel respected, he needs for you to show him your respect. BOTH in times when you are happy with him, AND when you are feeling frustrated.

5- Make Him Like A Winner He Wants To Be

- There is a certain truth to the statement that men are more in touch their minds while women are more in touch with their heart. In plain words, men are more "egoistic" than women. So most men want to feel manly and important; this becomes even more crucial for them in their relationships.

The way you make a guy feel like a winner is by oiling his ego, this might sound a little "manipulative" but men could care less if you "mean" it or you are "faking" it. They just get blinded when a woman adds a creamy layer of butter on their ego.

Men are quite wary of other men who try to "oil" their ego because they get a little suspicious of their intent but when a woman does it they just let their guard off. Making a guy feel like a winner and important because you love him and want him to feel more confident and proud.

You may also want to make your man feel important because he will then like to be in your company which is one of the secret of keeping a man. The male ego is a fragile one, Like women, men need to know you care, that you are appreciative and that you make them feel like a winner. Just as daily compliments and sweet kisses makes women feel feminine and pretty.

6- Let Him Feel He Is In Control Even If You Are

- A great deal of women these days respect the male authority in their relationships, and they want to keep the men in control to make decisions, though with equality, it can be difficult for a man to take charge sometimes, so girls like to make the man feel in control.

Here are a few things you can do to give your guy the reigns-

1. Prove His Value:

Men, by nature, need the approval of their woman to know that they are doing their jobs properly, and without this reassurance they feel weak and powerless. Make your guy feel in control by showing him what a great job he is doing of taking care of your needs.

2. Respect His Authority:

Just like everyone else, your man wants to know that he is right all the time, even when he isn't. Of course, he will be wrong every once in a while, but even then, if it is possible, let him know that you think he made the right decision and that you respect his power. This will help him feel in control and it will also let him know that you respect his authority.

3. Know How to Appreciate Him:

It is very important that you know how to give your guy

the compliments he needs. It will keep him happy and know that you do not take him for granted.

4. Show Him His Importance:

Your man needs to know how important he is in your sexual life, so make sure that you are surprising him and fulfilling his needs to make him feel in control.

5.Value His Opinion:

When you ask him for his advice, make sure you take it or at least heavily consider it. If he thinks that he has an important part in the decisions that you make, it will show him that he essentially holds the authority in your relationship.

6. Give Him Space :

A woman who is clingy and needy all of the time tends to drive a man away, and by giving him his space when he needs it, it gives him the feeling of power that he needs in the relationship. If you allow him to work on himself, he will feel like he is in power.

7. Love His Life:

Men have hobbies that many women do not appreciate, but if you try to involve yourself with his interests and his favorite activities, then you are showing him that his personal life is very important and he will feel in control.

7- Don't Try To Change Him Instead Show What He Stands To Gain If Makes The Change Himself

- Not all relationships reach the last stages, however, and oftentimes it's because you cannot overlook your partner's shortcomings any longer. Even his good points can start irritating you.

At such a time, you sincerely believe that they must change for the sake of you, their loved one, and of the relationship. If you want to keep your man the best thing is to forget about principles and to accept the man with all his pluses and minuses. If you are head over heels in love, then be ready to make concessions.

The thing you should accept is that it is fine to be different; your interests, goals, and characters make the relationship unique.

8- His Wired To Provide But Don't Push Him

- It's not the pain. It's not the fear. It's not the terrified hopelessness of losing him. It's that most of the time a woman's reaction to a man becoming distant will actually drive him away more and push him further and further away from her.

The typical reaction that many women have to a man becoming distant is one that actually works against her and makes him withdraw even more.so the best thing not to push him.

9- Be Happy, He Will Love You Even More

- The simplest and usually best way to keep a man around is to make him know you feel happy being with it, this would make him happy always. This doesn't mean giving him everything he says he wants, like things you're not comfortable with.

Instead, make your man feel happy by showing that you understand him, caring for him, and appreciating him for who he is. Being happy yourself doesn't hurt, either, since a loving man will love knowing how happy he makes you.

Ways to make your man happy:
Compliment him.
No matter what he says or how he acts about it, your boyfriend (like everyone else) appreciates hearing nice

things about himself. We all seek validation for how we look and what we do, especially when it comes from someone we care about. It's good for your boyfriend's ego, his pride, and his happiness.

10- Have Your Space And Give Him His

- Understand that it's okay to give your man space, The sooner you accept that it's normal, healthy, and absolutely necessary for a flourishing relationship, the better it'll be for the both of you.

If things have been reaching the breaking point in your relationship, try letting the situation go for a while. Don't try to control what he's doing or fixate on what you're not getting out of the relationship; when you let things be, they often have a way of fixing themselves.

Realize that your man is more likely to break up with you if you keep breathing down his neck than if you give him the space he craves.

11- Don't Cling But Show Him What He Stands To Lose If He Distances Himself

- If you want to show a man what he stands to lose if he distance himself you will have to stand up for yourself. No one is afraid of a weakling woman but a strong, empowered woman knows that she has to back up her word with actions and her punishment with actions. If you don't mean it he won't believe you, you have to be believable.

If you are terrified of losing him, no matter what he does to you how could you possibly expect him to have any fear of losing you whatsoever.when you show him you would stay with him at the expense of your own self respect, dignity and happiness he would never want to lose you and I repeat he would never want to lose you.

12- Set Your Boundaries, Keep He's And Enforce Them

- Creating healthy boundaries is empowering. By recognizing the need to set and enforce limits, you protect your self-esteem, maintain self-respect, and enjoy healthy relationships. Unhealthy boundaries cause emotional pain that can lead to dependency, depression, anxiety, and even stress-induced physical illness.

A lack of boundaries is like leaving the door to your home unlocked: anyone, including unwelcome guests, can enter at will. On the other hand, having too rigid boundaries can lead to isolation, like living in a locked-up castle surrounded by a mote.

No one can get in, and you can't get out. The easiest way to think about a boundary is a property line. We have all seen "No Trespassing" signs, which send a clear message that if you violate that boundary, there will be a consequence.

This type of boundary is easy to picture and understand because you can see the sign and the border it protects. Personal boundaries can be harder to define because the lines are invisible, can change, and are unique to each individual. Personal boundaries, just like the "No

Trespassing" sign, define where you end and others begin and are determined by the amount of physical and emotional space you allow between yourself and others. Personal boundaries help you decide what types of communication, behavior, and interaction are acceptable.

Boundaries are more than just lines on a map. In relationships, they are mandatory codes of conduct that need to be respected. It's where we draw the line on what is acceptable behavior and what is not.

13- Don't Manipulate Him

- Manipulation is a behavior in which one person tries to change the mind of another person without confronting them directly. Manipulators use deception, trickery and threats to get what they want, from people who are willing to give in to them. Now all of us don't fall for the tricks of a manipulator all the time.

But there are instances when all of us can fall prey to manipulation, especially when we're being used by someone we love and really care about. The easiest way to see it is by understanding the way you feel around a person.

When you feel powerless in the presence of someone, there's a good chance that you're being manipulated by them, whether you realize it or not! The first thing you need to understand is that people get manipulated, not because they're weak, but because they truly believe they stand to lose something by not giving in to this person.

And it's most common in romantic relationships where one partner always gives in to the other partner just to please them or to avoid offending them. Don't manipulate your man into something he dosen't want to be.

14- Don't Play Games

- No one would argue that dating is tough these days. But while we may refer to it as the dating game, games are the last thing you need if you want to find a man or if you want to keep the one you already have.

There are tons of "rules" that different "experts" have outlined in order for you to obtain or keep a man, and they usually involve playing some kind of manipulation. Having some sort of guide may seem comforting, but in fact it's counter-productive.

Playing games never works in love. The only thing dating has in common with a game are the elements of risk and chance. In order to have a healthy, successful, adult relationship, you have to stop playing games.

Reasons why you need to forfeit and allow yourself to live in the moment:

1. In relationships, there should be no winners or losers:

If your goal is always to win, you will always lose. If you're biggest concern is always having the upper hand, you most likely aren't in the headspace or at a maturity level to be in a real relationship.

Relationships thrive on vulnerability and being able to let your guard down. Playing games and "winning" a relationship should never be a game. While there's always a winner in chess, in a relationship if all you do is protect the queen (i.e. yourself), you'll surely find yourself without a king – maybe sooner than you think.

2. You're generally going against your gut.

Unless you're a manipulative sociopath, playing games is not your natural reaction or instinct about everything related to the opposite sex.

When you do this, you're ignoring your intuition for the sake of some rule you think you're supposed to follow about how long it should be before you text a guy back or whatever the case may be. We have a gut for a reason and when we ignore it, things rarely work out.

3. The law of attraction will work against you.

You're supposed to put out there what you want to receive back. If the only energy you're putting out into the universe with your relationships is disingenuous and interested in manipulation, guess what you're going to get back? Yep. Unless you have a weird mental fetish for game playing, you're only setting yourself up for disaster and heartbreak.

4. You're setting a dangerous precedent.

If you start playing games in the beginning, what sort of precedent are you setting for your relationship if it progresses? Come on, we've all heard Oprah: a relationship can't survive if you aren't being your authentic self, and what's less authentic than being underhanded?

Once you start playing games with a guy, where does it end? Will he play them back with you? What if he doesn't know the rules? What if he plays the game by different rules? And do you really want to be with a guy who plays games, too?

5. You aren't giving a guy the chance to fall for you.

If you're playing games with and attracting guys you're giving them the chance to get to know the you in the game. When you stop playing games, the attraction might not be there.

Maybe you guys thrived on the chaos of it all. Whenever you're presenting a false sense of self, you run the greater risk of your relationship not working when you finally let the guard down and are yourself.

6. Games become frustrating for all involved.

The thing about games – especially when they don't come with a pair of dice, board, and instruction book – is that the rules can change at any given time. Any player can change them, and anyone can quit whenever they want.

It can be difficult and frustrating to try to keep up with who's playing what game at what time and your partner could at some point throw in the towel on your relationship or what would've been your relationship. Doing this with a mate or potential mate could unintentionally have the opposite effect.

7. You can't manipulate love.
Love is fluid. It's an emotion. It involves two people who change and whose feelings change on a daily and even possibly an hourly basis. As much as you want to try to play games with a guy to try to minimize any potential risk your heart is taking, you can't.

As is evident with all of the earlier reasons you need to stop playing games, you can't manipulate love or people into falling in love or feeling the way you want them to feel. It's unfortunate, but if you like a guy, you're going to have to just buckle up and get ready for the ride.

8. There really is beauty in an unforeseen future.
If you knew that a guy would give you butterflies on Tuesday at 4pm, the feeling wouldn't be as precious, would it? If you knew that you were going to have a massive fight but the world's best makeup sex two weeks from tomorrow, life would be pretty boring, right?

As much as it's uncomfortable to live in the moment and be vulnerable and put yourself out there, you can't be in a real relationship if you don't. Instead of fighting it, try to find the beauty in the not knowing and the unexpected.

You will probably get your heart broken but you will also have some amazing surprises in store for you that wouldn't be as magical if you knew they were coming around the corner.

15- Be Supportive Even When He Falls Shot
 • The best possible thing you can get out of a relationship

is that you're with someone who encourages you to be the best version of yourself every day. If you look at any relationship which has lasted a long time, you will find that it is generally a supportive relationship.

A supportive relationship is a relationship which brings mutual benefit to both parties helping them to cope with the tough times and maximise the good times. Simply put, a supportive relationship enables you to achieve more than you ever could on your own.

16- Constructively Criticize Tenderly

- When you're in a serious relationship you're constantly learning about yourself, your partner, and the things that make you soar, stagnate, or crumble. Over time you can learn how to have difficult conversations together with your partner so you can attack and face problems straight on so things don't fester.

Don't have these types of conversations if you just had a fight and either of you are feeling angry or agitated. Tell your significant other you need to be alone for an hour or two to cool off first. Before you have a serious conversation with each other, take the time to reflect on what is bothering you, and what is bothering your partner.

They are probably completely different things. Remember, for every issue you want to coach your significant on, think of several skills or tasks they've done well and BREATHE between each sentence.

17- Show Him You Can Be Independent

- An independent woman is her own person. This may sound similar to the first point, but it functions differently. Such a trait is displayed more when you first meet a person but is applicable in a long-term relationship. Being your own person means being willing to stand up for yourself and have your own opinions.

I often hear from female friends they may not enjoy or agree with certain things a boyfriend or potential suitor says, but they refuse to say anything because they don't want to offend him and risk "scaring him away."

A woman in a relationship should have more priorities than just her boyfriend. This could be work, school, a social life anything that allows her to be her own person and have a life away from her boyfriend.

This is important not just because it gives the guy more time to be with his friends (though it helps), but because it allows both parties to focus and give all their attention to each other when they do spend time with one another.

For example, when were in school; my girlfriend and I attend different universities and we both did this on purpose. It may seem counter-intuitive to want to be apart from one another, but the reasoning is that we need to keep certain aspects of our life separate.

Men tend to operate more on this principle than women do, but it does make sense. When you keep your worlds separate, you can give each one the focus and attention it deserves.

18- Be Available But Not Overly Available

- Availability, in the dating context, means how available you are to him when he seeks any form of contact. This includes but is not limited to, how often you respond to his phone calls, how often and how quickly you text him back, how willing you are to engage in text/e-mail/facebook/etc.

Conversation, adding him to social networks, being

available when he wants to meet up in person, and the like. As I hinted earlier, the reason availability matters is because it is correlated to desperation and neediness.

It is also correlated to investment which I wrote about here. The more available you are, particularly for non-romantic activities, the more needy and desperate you may appear. If you demand something in return for availability, and demand some availability on his part, you make him invest. There is of course, a balance. The main risk of being too available is coming off as needy and or too interested.

For this reason, it is important not to be too available unless he is already interested. Once you "got him", once he is interested, you have less to worry about regarding appearing needy. You still don't want to be available for hour long phone calls every night (especially if you aren't getting laid, and even if you are), but you don't have to "play games.

19- Men Sometimes Can Behave Like Little Boys But Never Treat Them As Such

- If your man sometimes behave or act like a little boy the best way to deal with this is to treat him as if he were as old as he's acting. He wants to pout? Fine. He can do that. Doesn't mean you have to deal with it. Go do something else until he's ready to act his age.

20- Sexy And Brains All Rolled Into One Are The Ultimate Turn-Ons For Men

- Intelligent people have so many layers to them, so it takes time to get to know them. But one thing is guaranteed: peeling away those layers will leave you wanting more. Someone who's able to blow your mind by picking your brain can be so much more attractive than someone who obsesses over their appearance.

We learn to love them for what they most love about

themselves. You bond over your favorite books and deepest beliefs and honest conversations. The whole process of getting to know them is a sexy geek fest of your favorite quotes and the artists nobody else knows.

You love being able to understand and figure out what your partner loves. You're exposed to ideas and writing and art that you never before would have come across or maybe even appreciated, and it's in that moment that you end up giving to one another so much more than just your time and attention.

When you date an intelligent person, you're loved for the person you are, beyond what you appear to be, or the physical space you inhabit. It's what everybody claims to want, yet so few people know how to achieve.

People attracted to intelligence inherently understand that we are more than our bodies. They understand they are temporary, both in lifespan and in taut, smooth, young attractiveness. You're seen and desired for who you most genuinely are.

21- Get Your Timing Right In Handling Situations

- One cannot truly love until he learns to love himself. You may have heard this phrase, or some derivative of it, at least once before. And while it is a statement whose meaning bares all truth, there is another factor that can obliterate the already tainted tenor of love: timing. The truth is, there is never a perfect or ideal time to initiate a relationship.

Of course, the stability of one relies on the proper balance of mental and emotional conditions of both parties. However, waiting for one person to be completely content in the mind, body and heart simultaneously is useless.

Expecting such conditions from two people simultaneously is even more absurd. For a relationship to function thoroughly you don't need perfect conditions; what you do need is to be familiar with them.

This is where the false accusation of timing comes into the picture. Many say that if they are undergoing distressing circumstances in their lives, they cannot commit to someone else. And that makes perfect sense.

You should never put someone else's happiness above your own, and as mama always said, you have to make sure your room is clean before you can go play in someone else's. The mistake people make when they acknowledge the "bad timing" is oversimplifying the meaning of a relationship.

Having a partner to share your experiences with isn't a job and should never be a daunting task. It isn't about calling and checking in every night or kissing your girlfriend's ass so that she would trust you. Nor is it about frequent dinner dates and excuses to spend your money.

Those things can and, under the right circumstances, should be done, but they don't define the relationship. A relationship should, above all things, be two people sharing their lives as partners, experiencing it as friends and enjoying it as lovers.

Any protocol, any standard relationship etiquette- anything that comes from the outside of that relationship should immediately be disregarded. With that being said, if you're at a low point in your life but you have someone that, under better circumstances, would be your significant other, they can still be in your life.

If they care for you and you are, in fact, right for each

other, the relationship mumbo jumbo can be put on hold. They will understand your inability to commit at that specific point, but they will still be there for you.

The timing in this situation is bad in the sense that you're not completely content with yourself at that given moment. That doesn't mean the timing has to put a strain on your relationship. If your partner cares for you and your wellbeing, they'll give you the time and space you need to recover- unless, of course, you make the mistake of pushing them away.

In which case, it wasn't timing that did you wrong, but instead the way you handled your distressing circumstances and the current situation. Another mistake people make when claiming the "timing is wrong" is putting the wrong offender to blame.

They put the emphasis on the wrong words. Is the timing wrong because you're not ready to commit to them or are you not ready to commit to them? It's very possible that your inability to enter a relationship isn't because of where you are in your life, but rather whom you are with.

At this time you have to be 100% honest with yourself. If you have lingering doubts about someone that were brought to light through no other outside cause, it's probably not meant to be. If anything would make you hesitate as such, it's doubt.

When the right person comes into your life, you're supposed to just know. Which leads us to the next mistake people make. What if you just don't know? There is one and only one instance where timing qualifies as a legitimate excuse. Stress in your life and doubts are separate factors that corrupt your relationships, but they do not hide under the signature of time.

22- Focus On What He Does Not What He Says

- If you've ever heard the saying, "actions speak louder than words", understand that this sentiment rings true when it comes to love as well. When a man truly loves a woman, his actions will be extremely difficult to ignore.

When questioning the love of a man for YOU, consider these eight actions to get the answer:

1. He calls:

When a man loves you, he makes the effort to regularly call you. He wants to know how your day went, how you are feeling, and how he can make things better. This concept of going days without speaking isn't synonymous with a man who really loves a woman. When he's really in love, he has to force himself not to call every day because it's instinctual.

2. He finds ways to touch:

Men express their love through physical touch. While many women love physical touch as well, they respond to emotional touch more. However, men naturally love to look at and touch the woman they love. This touch doesn't necessarily equate to love-making. Simple taps on the back, playful touch, or a simple high-five are ways he shows his love through touch.

3. He helps:

If there's ever a time when a woman needs help with a certain situation, the man will be there to help in any way he can. For the man who's really in love, his woman's needs come before his own. If he knows she's hungry, he's going to do what he needs to do to find food for her.

4. He sticks around:

One of the most common traits of a healthy

relationship involves conflict. Even though conflict can be uncomfortable, it is important for building intimacy and strengthening communication skills. Unfortunately, at the mere thought of a fight, many guys run. The man who's in love won't run. He'll stick around and work through it because the woman he loves is worth it.

5. He yields:

Another common component of a healthy relationship is the ability to compromise. There are many ways compromise shows up in a relationship. Compromise might involve going to see one movie instead of another. It could mean going to see one set of parents at Thanksgiving and the other at Christmas. Either way, compromise is important for any family.

6. He makes plans:

A man who's in love will make plans to see his woman. He has a hard time foreseeing the future without her and as a result, he begins to build her into his life. A man who's not in love will merely suggest things at a moment's notice. Adequate planning doesn't go into the enjoyment of their lives together when a man's not in love.

7. He introduces family:

People love to shout it out from the rooftops when they experience deep, real, passionate, exciting love. The man who's in love will at least share it with his family (let alone the world). This is primarily because in many cases, a man's family is his world.

8. He speaks the love language:

Every woman has a specific love language. Whether she enjoys gifts, words of affirmation, quality time, acts of service, or physical touch, a man in love will work to find out which one it is and overwhelm his woman with love. He wants her to understand the depth of his love for her in a way she can truly understand.

23- Remind Him Who He Is And Where He Wants To Be But Don't Lose Yourself Along The Way

- The only relationships that last are those that continue to grow and develop towards each person's individual goals. Once you realised you have lost touch with the dreams he once had, he becomes unhappy.

Those women who do their best to keep their lover's goals as the goals of the relationship as a unit are those who remain happiest and remain together the longest.

Luckily, the simplest form of helping your partner achieve their dreams is by facilitating the right type of environment for them. Like all things worth doing, making things work will require a bit of planning and discussion on individual priorities sharing our goals with the other and establishing a strong understanding of what it is that we need out of life.

It may seem a bit over the top, but if you have made it to the point in your relationship when you are beginning to seriously visualize a future together, then it's as good a time as any to actually consider the logistics of your future situation.

This talk should not be rushed because let's be honest it's a serious talk and could push your partner away rather than bring you closer together. But when the time does come, sit them down and ask them about their long-term and short-term goals.

Go into the projected path that your love plans on following and go into as much detail as possible. The more you know, the better you will be able to help your partner reach his goals. Prioritize and make your next goals (yours and theirs) clear as well as what role the other should play.

By not losing yourself along the line making him who he needs to be remember your man's goals are still his goals, not yours; and it must remain that way. What makes goals worth having is the journeyed traveled along the way.

If you butt in too much, you'll end up taking that away from them. Think of yourself as an on-call advisor or assistant. You give advice only when asked for it and lend a helping hand under the same circumstances. There are instances when your man will ask you to be more hands on, but keep in mind that you are doing this for him and not for your own personal gain.

24- Show Him You Are Not Perfect And You Don't Expect Him To Be Either

- He's not perfect. You aren't either, and the two of you will never be perfect. But if you can make him laugh at least once, causes him to think twice, and if he admits to being human and making mistakes, hold onto him and give him the most you can.

He isn't going to quote poetry, he's not thinking about you every moment, but he will give you a part of him that he knows you could break. Don't hurt him, don't change him, and don't expect more than he can give.

Don't analyze. Smile when he makes you happy, yell when he makes you mad, and miss him when he's not there. Love hard when there is love to be had. Because perfect guys don't exist, but there's always one guy that is perfect for you.

25- Show Him You Accept Agreeing To Disagree

- Even in the strongest of relationships, there will be times when small irritations can cause mountains to grow out of molehills, so it's important to keep striving for better communication. As the essence of relationships, communication has a great impact on every aspect of life.

Yet the channels of communication can sometimes become blocked, even among people who care deeply for each other. It's often difficult to put our feelings into words or concentrate fully when our partner speaks.

Unhelpful silences or verbal attacks can arise and drive us further apart. Common barriers to communication include: threatening or unpleasant behavior such as criticism and bossiness; only hearing what we want to hear; getting bored or distracted; and not expressing our point clearly.

Fortunately, working on our communication skills helps us to break through this sort of impasse. So follow these tried and tested tips to stop you reaching for the expletives and reach an understanding instead.

No matter what else is going on, try to make time for your partner on a day-to-day basis. Good communication is about deepening your understanding of each other, not simply avoiding arguments.

Easier said than done, of course, but making time to talk is worth the effort. All being well, these occasions will be enjoyable and bring great rewards, so make a dinner date, share a bath or go for a walk together and let the conversation flow.

Secondly, remember the importance of intimate, non-sexual contact. Hugs and kisses are the glue which holds a relationship together, and consider activities such as sport to reconnect non-verbally. Psychologists believe the vast majority of communication takes place without words through body language.

Do you believe you know everything there is to know about your partner? It may be worth checking this out by asking them questions to reveal more about themselves. To deepen the communication and understanding between you, try talking about the times when you feel happiest or your hopes and dreams for the future.

Don't assume that your partner feels the same way you do. This could bring up relationship 'hot spots' – work, money, childcare – which can then be dealt with openly. Experts suggest setting up reciprocal arrangements in which you both agree to take on an equal number of tasks and chores.

If you find yourself slipping into an argument, there are many ways to keep the row healthy. Most importantly, own your emotions by using "I" statements. For example, rather than "You make me angry," or "This is all your fault," try saying, "I feel concerned/upset…".

This keeps things calmer and makes it easier to compromise, as your partner will not become so defensive. Then keep to the point rather than slipping into attack and counter-attack, or emotional withdrawal. But talking this way is only possible if you are aware of your own feelings.

For this, you must recognize them, be accepting of them, and able to express them. We each have our own way of dealing with conflicts – your style may be to avoid the issue, give in, or blame the other person.

Being aware of your style and that of your partner will help you resolve the situation. In the heat of the moment, try to stay calm and accentuate the positive. See the other's point of view while showing respect, and then look for a compromise that you can both accept.

Listen carefully, give empathy and positive responses, and overlook the insults. Respond to criticism as useful information, if at all possible! Remember, the objective is not to stop every argument but to stop the escalating bitterness. If either partner gets beyond the point of being civil and rational, ask for a "time-out" to calm down.

But be sure to agree on continuing the discussion when you have had time to think about it. Bear in mind that one of the secrets of happy couples is learning to tolerate or accept the other person's faults.

So-called "perfect relationships" do not exist, therefore small faults need to be accepted. Couples counseling encourages reaching an acceptance of one another through compassion and empathy, so you both come to truly understand the other person and become able to share your own feelings in depth.

Then you can see the underlying reasons for their criticism or silence, perhaps they are really feeling unloved, rejected or hurt. Having awareness of these techniques and skills is only half the battle – you need to develop them through practice until they become second nature.

It will be an effort to change long-standing habits, but improving communication in your relationship is worth doing, as poor communication is one of the top causes of unhappy relationships.

26- Be Honest And Expect Same From Him

- Can you really tell a man everything on your mind even the not-so-pretty stuff? Yes as long as you know these critical elements about how to communicate with him first. Has a man ever told you of some plans he had to hang out with his friends, or travel somewhere by himself for whatever reason, and you pretended to be perfectly okay with it because you didn't want to seem "needy?"

But then later, when he came back! All those hurt, angry feelings came out, he withdrew, and then there's a wedge between the two of you. You might conclude that you can't be honest with a man, when in reality a little tweaking in terms of timing and delivery can make all the difference, Here's something you may not know about men, or even agree with, but it's true.

A man absolutely wants you to be honest and straight-forward with him. This is what men like so much about the way they can communicate with each other. And, in fact, it drives them nuts when you aren't open and direct.

If they are planning something that you don't agree with, they want you to let them know at the start – as soon as possible – before it becomes a bigger issue or concern. Here's the beauty of telling a man what you think early on: it allows you to communicate in a way that's less combative and negative than it would be if you were to have it fester in your mind for a while.

27- Show Him Your Vulnerable Side But Let Him Understand You Can't Be Taken Advantage Of

- Let's define "taking for granted" for the purpose of everyone being on the same page. Taking someone for granted is when a person is not appreciating something or someone for what they are, have to offer or are doing for them.

It is when one's actions or presence is not valued in the relationship. I believe when someone is taking us granted, it is of primary importance to first sit down to a conversation about it- vulnerable, raw and real.

I believe the due process of all relationship matters is to share all grievances openly so that a dialogue can begin. In this, we are coming from our Highest Self (not our fearful, hiding, assuming self). We have already taken the higher road by not assuming our partner is doing this on purpose or already knows what he/she is doing.

It is important to choose Right Speech (clear, loving, non-emotional) when discussing any matter. Focus on using "I feel" statements rather than attack statements like: You never blank blank blank! Attack from one person usually leads to defense and counter-attack from another.

Keep the conversation open and progressive. it is time to tell him again, but this time with your actions and behavior. Whatever area you feel you are being taken for granted for, stop doing! Sound too simple?

Well, it is that simple! When you take the gesture away, he will either begin to notice and appreciate the work/time/love you were putting into the partnership or he won't notice at all (perhaps because it wasn't a big deal for him, but more so for you).

With that, you will either begin to get the appreciation and respect you deserve or you will have just freed up valuable time to focus on something else of your choosing. In my opinion, either way it's a win! Remember, all change in relationship starts with you.

Be willing to step forward, dialogue about the subject and change your behavior if needed. This is how we stay empowered. If you are feeling taken for granted in your relationship, the first thing to do is to look at your own behavior, Decide if you are showing your partner enough love, affection and affirmation.

This can be done by welcoming them home, giving hugs and kisses regularly, reaching for their hand, sending thoughtful text or email messages, leaving little love notes in cute spots and regularly complimenting them.

If you are showing your partner plenty of affirmation then it is time to tactfully request what you need. Let your partner know that you are feeling taken for granted and give your partner a variety of ideas that will make you feel important and loved. A caring partner should start adding a few small gestures into their daily routine.

28- Flirt With Him But Let Him Feel He Is The One That Initiated It

- One of the most important things to know before flirting with your man is to let him know you're warm and approachable, and a girl who wouldn't mind a bit of flirting. Guys may think twice before trying to flirt with girls, but if you follow these ten tips on how to flirt him and you would make him feel he is the one that initiated it, And you know this little secret, don't you?

Guys are drawn and attracted to a girl they can flirt with. So use these ten tips on flirting with a guy and work your magic, girl! Remember, you don't ever have to make the first move if you know these tips on how to flirt with a guy.

Just follow these steps, and you can make any guy you like flirt with you without ever making the first move

1. Smile, blush and be coy:

Guys love a girl who's happy and full of positivity. And guys especially love a girl who smiles and laughs when she's having a conversation with them. Don't be arrogant, rude or pass cocky comments when you're with the guy you want to flirt with.

Guys stay away from girls who behave this way, even if they're attractive looking. Be warm and approachable, and have a nice time when you're talking to a guy. Smile a lot and blush when he compliments you, and we assure you his heart will skip a beat!

2. Compliment him and thank him:
Guys love compliments, and compliments are one of the stepping stones of a happy flirty conversation. If you like something about a guy, make sure you compliment him for that. He would love the fact that you noticed something nice about him, and furthermore, he'd go out of his way to have a flirty conversation with you.

And likewise, if he's being rather courteous or chivalrous, thank him with a warm smile. When you acknowledge a guy's chivalry or gestures positively, he'll try harder to please you. And along the way, he'll be warmer and will flirt more, just to win your attention.

3 . Stare into his eyes:
One of the secrets of knowing how to flirt with a guy is to indulge in everything that someone in love does. You don't really need to be in love with him to win his heart, you just need to be happy and excited to be with him.] The next time you're having a conversation with a guy you like, look into his eyes deeply and smile as he's talking to you. It may confuse him or make him feel awkward, but a deep eye contact and a happy smile will definitely leave him weak in his knees.

4. Be expressive:
Have you ever seen Nigella Lawson on her show? She may be over fifty, but that woman can have any guy on his knees with just her feminine, flirty expressions. Spend a few

minutes in front of the mirror every day and work on your expressions.

Learn to use your eyes and your facial expressions to your advantage, and you won't really need words to impress a guy and make him flirt with you. Learn to flutter your eyelids, work your smile and your little happy expressions, and va-va-voom! You'll be a flirty goddess no guy can ignore or deny.

And if you're wondering if expressions can really make a difference, do you really think women like Angeline Jolie, Elisha Cuthbert and Brande Roderick were born with those awe inspiring flirty expressions? It may take a few weeks or months, but learning to use your expressions to your advantage can change your life forever.

5. Do that thing with your hair:
Now don't ask us why, but guys are suckers for great hair. Perhaps, it's because they can't play flirty with their hair like women can. But guys love it when women run their hands through their hair.

The next time you're in the middle of a conversation, you can run your hands through your hair to show off your confidence or tuck your hair behind your ears with your fingers to show off your sexy cuteness. But whatever you do, it'll only make a guy's jaw drop in awe.

6 .Tease him:
If you really want to know how to flirt with a guy, you should also learn to put him down in jest, or make him work harder to impress you. You can't always put him on a pedestal using happy words. If his joke isn't really funny, say it.

If he's trying too hard, say it. Pull a guy down a few

notches once in a while, and he'll only overdo himself to prove himself to you. Always remember this, if you want to successfully flirt with a guy and make him like you, you have to make him feel special.

But the flirty game still has to be in your control. You should make him feel nice, but teasing him in jest or putting him down once in a rare while gives him something to fight for. You know how competitive men are, use it against him and he'll only try harder.

7. Don't be loud or brash:

Almost all manly guys with raging testosterones like a girly girl. You don't need to act like a dainty princess out of a fairy tale all the time, but when you're having a conversation with a guy, try to be subtle and feminine, be it in your voice or the way you dress. This may seem rude, but a brash or loud girl is actually more of a turn off for guys than anything else.

8. Touch him now and then:

This is one of the best ways to make a guy desire you and want to flirt with you. Men just can't help but go weak in the knees when a girl they're flirting with, touches them.

It's involuntary, but every time a girl touches a guy, either on his arm or his shoulder, the guy opens up more and feels more comfortable to talk to the girl or flirt with her. Learn to touch a guy now and then while talking to him and you'll see how easy it will be to make him flirt with you in minutes!

9. Be girly:

You don't have to act like a school girl to win a guy's heart, but if you want a guy to start flirting with you, you need to make him feel like he can protect you. Men have always been the hunters and the protectors through evolution.

So if you want him to be drawn to you, you need to let him take the lead at least for a few minutes. Men like to take the lead, be it asking a girl out or flirting with her, so just play it easy and wait for him to start flirting with you.

After all, you don't want to start flirting before he does and risk a chance of getting blown off, do you? And, something to think about if you were in the sitcom, Community, do you think it would be easier to flirt with Britta or Annie? As annoying as it may seem, you do know what works with guys now, don't you.

10. Make him feel special:
If you've understood how to flirt with a guy, you'd know how important it is to make a guy you're flirting with feel special. Now, you don't need to do anything new here, but you need to remember that when you make a guy feel special, he'd get attracted to you and would want to be with you.

Make him feel special with your smile and your expressions, and your compliments and your flirty touches, and any guy you like would want to flirt with you and would find you desirable in no time.

29- Show Him The Door To Your Heart But Let Him Work To Get In

- To be loved as much as your heart's deepest desire, you have to open yourself to love, and love in return. Open your heart even when your memories from the past guard you. There may have been many men who were not worthy of your trust.

But there will be one who is. And if you're fortunate, you may have been able to trust all the men you have been with.

And every time you feel like closing down yet feel your man's longing for intimacy with you, his advances towards you choose first to understand him.

And then understand yourself, and realize your full capacity as a feminine woman to open fully and unguarded to him. Again, it doesn't have to be sex. But the more you open, and the more you are in sync with your man, the less you will want to resist him. IF he is worthy of you as a woman.

The greatest gift a woman can be given by a worthy man is to be polarized by his masculine energy of direction, integrity and passion. This makes it easy for you to go in to your feminine core again. The problem is, that if you have a man who is more in his feminine, you'll be depolarized, and you'll be forced to find your way, and make your own direction.

To lead yourself – and you'll probably even find yourself leading the relationship. And the less loved and appreciated you feel, the more you'll want to retreat; to close off your deepest source of love, and your deepest desire for love and intimacy. And, I'm not going to lie, women are great leaders. Sometimes you'll have to, even if and when it feels unnatural to you.

If you're a part of the corporate world, you'll be doing it at work all day. But in relationship, you need to allow yourself to be polarized. The less you feel a man's direction, the more you'll want to do your best to lead yourself. And him.

And everything else This is the exact position many women are in today. But by opening, by being inviting, you'll invite and encourage more of his presence and masculinity. And in turn, feel your own freedom.

30- Don't Be Judgmental

- If you don't like something he said say it but don't create a huge ruckus over it .The guy may have different tastes then you and he may like doing things that you don't but that does not allow you to insult him for it.

Show a genuine interest in what he is saying ,share your opinions also but don't be rude or judgemental. The ability to discern what we like or dislike is an important part of being an individual. It is enriching to have choices about what to eat, what we like to wear, how to decorate our space, or what our favorite movie is.

Many of our choices become part of how we define ourselves. Some of our self-definitions go deeper and concern whether we prefer to be open about our emotions. If we came from a family in which emotions were not talked about, we will most likely be less inclined to talk about emotions.

Another person may have grown up in a family in which emotions were expressed openly and honestly. If two people from such different families establish a romantic relationship, problems may arise.

While it's important for all of us to have choices as individuals, it's equally important for partners to be tolerant of each other's differences. This is especially true during the early years of a partnership, when partners typically work together to define how they want their own family to be.

The early years of a relationship are often about building a new family that is different from either partner's family of origin. If one partner becomes judgmental and critical of the other partner's way of being, problems generally ensue.

Judgment often leads a person to become contemptuous of the other person, and contempt is hard to conceal. We all have micro-expressions that cross our faces so quickly we may not even know we have expressed the feelings associated with them.

One's partner might see those micro-expressions and feel deeply hurt by them. The most important skill in any close relationship is the ability to understand and empathize. Empathy is the opposite of contempt, disgust, or other negative judgment.

The way to empathy is through understanding, and judgment blocks understanding. Understanding a person takes a lot more intellectual and emotional work than judgment does. True understanding comes from active listening and appreciation of what the other person is trying to convey.

True understanding comes from realizing that our own way of being is just that our own way and not everybody will want to be as we are. If you try to listen to, appreciate, and understand another person's position but find you cannot, it may be that you need to recognize that your own way of thinking may be preventing you from relating well to that person.

Your way of thinking and being is different from his or her way of thinking and being. Can you accept that? Can you accept that a person you believe you love or care about is different from you in some ways? It is possible to love not only a person but his or her differences, too.

In fact, true, deep, and lasting love involves a great deal of acceptance of another's differences. Accepting a person's differences helps you become a better-rounded, happier, more likable, more trustworthy, more mature individual.

Maturity is not something that happens to us as we get older.

Maturity is something we gain through self-awareness, self-confrontation, and genuine efforts to grow and become kinder, more accepting, and at peace with other ways of being than your own.

31- Punish Him When He Is Cocky While Smiling

- If you are the kind of girl who forgives her guy even if he keeps her waiting then change that attitude. Don't let a guy take you for granted.When you are getting into a relationship it is imperative that he takes you seriously.

Ignore him if he throws his weight or gives more attention to someone else and scold him also if necessary. Do this at the beginning of the relationship but only when he takes you for granted .The rest of time you should be the sweetest girl around him.

32- If You Win A Debate Don't Rob It In

- Men stay in awe of a woman who is intelligent .Never let the guy feel he is more intelligent then you.Be aware of the current affairs and talk to him about it .When a guy feels you are unintelligent he will treat you as his arm candy and not as his life partner.

33- Be Naughty But Not Overtly

- Women can find a bunch of tips out there on the internet on pleasing your man and being a better lady for him, but most of the advice out there is missing the essence. You have to focus on pushing the right buttons in your guys mind so that he'll literally go mad of excitement once he orgasms. As a result, your man will love you more than ever.

So the thing is get naughty, Really naughty but not overtly. Guys want you to be "dirty" in bed, and an angel in front of their mother. So do exactly that. A lot of you ladies are afraid that their man will think low of them, well he won't.

On the contrary, he'll adore you for being his personal porn star in bed. Why do you think men watch pornography? Think about it. 95% of guys out there want you to be naughty, sexual, daring. Nobody wants a robot girlfriend in bed that's afraid of opening up and letting go.

Get comfortable with that guy, start feeling good in your body. That leads to the second thing you should do to drive him mad.

34- Be Approachable

- Contrary to what you may think, getting hit on or appearing approachable to men isn't really a game of chance where you just have to wait it out. And contrary to what most women think, you don't have to do something outrageous or provocative to get a guy to walk up to you and say hello!

The truth is, if you understand a guy's mind and what goes on in it before he approaches a girl, you could make any guy want to strike up a conversation with you within five minutes of stepping into a place.

First and foremost, you have to remember that guys are human, too. They may come across as cocky and arrogant. They may seem like womanizers from the outset, but really they too have fears about being the one to approach women they find attractive.

Of course, there are some super confident guys out there who will take the initiative and approach the women they're attracted to, but the majority won't. Why? If a man is really interested in you and not looking for a one night stand there's always going to be the fear of rejection looming at the back of his mind.

Just like you, he too doesn't want to be disappointed or embarrassed by being turned down. Sometimes, without even realizing it, women do not do themselves any favors. Sometimes they just don't get that what they're doing and that how they're acting is actually repelling guys and not attracting them.

The key here is to open up a little more and try and make yourself more approachable. There are some things that you're doing that guys view as standoffish. So, pay careful attention and learn ways to make yourself warmer and easier to talk to.

And just so you know, despite what every woman seems to think, you don't have to do anything provocative or outrageous to get a man's attention.

Here's how to be more approachable:

1. Appearance Matters:
This in no way means that you have to be the next Kate Moss or Gisele Bündchen. You don't have to have supermodel good looks or be a size zero, but you do need to look good and take care of yourself.

It's shallow, I know, but the first impression you give a person is always through how you look. When a guy enters a room, it doesn't take him long to notice the women he finds physically attractive.

If you take care of your appearance by keeping your hair neat, your clothes tidy, you're your makeup simple and natural, you're going to boost your chances of getting a guy to approach you.

2. Don't Busy Yourself:

If you spot a guy checking you out and you happen to be alone, don't make yourself look like you're completely engrossed in something such as sending an email on your iPad or reading your book.

It's quite possible that you're bored out of brain and just trying to pass some time before you have to head back to work or meet a friend, but this can be detrimental to meeting someone new. You'll appear too "busy" and, if he's a polite guy, he's not going to want to interrupt you.

3. You're Out of His League:

This totally goes against my first tip about looking the part. However, we have to be realistic because there's also a major drawback: You might be too good looking for a particular guy – i.e. You're out of his league.

For example, if you're an absolute stunner all the guys who pass you by are most likely going to drool over you from a distance and try to steal a few looks, but realistically the majority of guys are going to feel too intimidated by your great looks and not approach you at all – it's a catch-22 situation.

One of a guy's biggest fears when approaching any woman is the fear of rejection and embarrassment. If you're drop-dead gorgeous, many guys will simply assume that you're out of their league and that they aren't worthy of your attention. Simply put, if you're too hot, you're also going to scare the guys away.

The guys you will attract are those Alpha males, the super confident ones, and let's not forget the players. If you're really intent on catching the eye of a shy man who seems nice, you need to make yourself more approachable.

Be a little bit friendlier, be warm and don't forget to smile.

4. It's in Your Eyes:
Smiling young couple holding hands and looking at each other at table, If you spot a guy who catches your eye and you see him checking you out, check him out, too. Glance at him from time to time and make sure you lock eyes with him.

Don't do it too much or you may freak him out, but your eye contact with him shows you're interested in him. You can show a guy in two ways that you're interested through eye contact. You can give him a quick glance, but slow look away or you can glance at him slowly.

Look at him casually, lock eyes for a second or two and give him a small smile. This will show that you're confident and you'll also let him know that you're interested at the same time. And read our article on how to use your eyes to get a guy to approach you.

5. Make it Easier:
Guys freak out when they see a girl they like enclosed by a big group of girls. A man will never approach a girl when she's surrounded by a number of her friends because it's intimidating. You have to make it a little easier for him. So, if you want to meet more men and be approached by them, you either need to spend some more time alone or with just one girlfriend.

6. Choose Where You Hang:
Not every place that you go creates the ideal setting for striking up of casual conversations. You want men to approach you, right? Then pick a perfect spot for casual conversations. The place doesn't need to be completely private. It does, however, have to be a place where not every busybody is going to turn their head in your direction and

check out what's happening. Places like coffee shops, book stores and libraries make for the perfect first-meet – the opportunity for conversations are limitless (that is if you're doing everything else right to be approachable).

7. Say "Cheese!":

No one likes to see an uptight person. A person who walks around like they've got the weight of the world on their shoulders is going to come across as unfriendly. The trick is to appear warm and happy – you'll look friendlier, which means you'll appear more approachable, too. If you look like a likeable person, you have more chance of catching a man's eye.

8 .Be Positive:

Beauty portrait of a young brunette woman with beautiful smile We all have crap days sometimes, but the key is to have fun. You need to come across as a positive person wherever you may be.

It's all down to the laws of attraction – positivity draws positivity; therefore, a happy woman will attract a happy guy. When you think about it, you'd never approach someone if he or she looked boring, right? Make yourself more interesting and be positive.

35- Don't Be Too Predictable, Keep Him Guessing Once In While

- Being predictable does two things in a relationship which should be avoided: Makes you easily managed by others who know how you'll react, and Makes you boring. Neither is good for relationships whether personal or professional.so it is better to be unpredictable and keep your man guessing ones in a while.

36- Show Him He's Got Competition In Other Guys

- Despite the evolutionary fact that men are competitive

by nature, you might be surprised to learn that relationship ready men don't always like competition, especially when there is a high probability of losing.

Contrary to popular belief, competition is actually more of a stressor for men than an ego-driven match. While men are definitely hunters when it comes to getting women in bed, such competitiveness might actually be a turn off to a relationship ready man as it may cause him to question how serious the woman is about finding a relationship if she's dating several men at a time.

Some ego-driven men might see the competition as a challenge, but most men will just see it as a waste of time.

A man's reaction to competition is loosely based on three factors: the woman herself, the level of connection he has with her and his level of interest in this woman. In general, if a man really likes a woman, his competitive nature will start to kick in and he'll want to stake claim on his territory, so to speak.

However, if a man isn't particularly interested in a woman, or if she's too hard to get, then it's not really worth the effort to him to continue to pursue her.

37- Ask For His Help But Don't Use Him
- Admit it or not, Men used to get so frustrated because you wouldn't ask for help when so obviously you needed it. Some women think that a man would get upset when she asked him to make her a meal or empty the dishwasher, or whatever, because she couldn't. if he loves you much he would definitely wants to help.

38- Seek His Protection But Don't Act Spineless
- Testosterone instills in a man the intense desire to be a winner. If a man fought hard to get a desirable and

elusive woman, he cannot stand for other men to win her as well. Imagine winning a gold medal in the Olympics, feeling like the ultimate winner and then seeing you neighbour, your best friend, your colleague and the retarded kid across the street win the same medal.

You would not feel like much of a winner anymore, would you? A man who admires a sense of dignity in his woman and considers her to be very sought after feels the urge to guard her to protect both her honor and his own status as a winner.

It is very exciting for a man to feel the need to guard and the more testosterone driven a man is, the more he thrives on competing and winning. At the same time, it is intensely depressing for a man to compete and lose. If a man sees himself as unable to win you from other men, he may refrain from trying if he is afraid he may lose.

This can even happen in a married man who reluctantly or even enthusiastically resigns himself to the role of the cuckold. His fear of losing stops him from competing. Alternatively, he may go rogue, cheat in this game and win by foul play. The overly controlling man is as fearful of competition as the overly permissive man.

A healthy man of honor and courage welcomes competition if he is likely to win. He enters the arena well prepared. Every man who is honorable has the natural inclination to guard his woman.

On one hand, this urge promotes chivalrous behaviour that makes a woman feel treasured. On the other hand, it can be oppressive and make a woman feel unfree. Like with all the values, the key is balancing it with other values.

A man who has respect for a woman, as a person and not

just a trophy, who cares deeply about her feelings will want her to have enough freedom to be happy. Another thing that tempers his need to control is trust.

If a man met his woman while she was out dancing with her friend, getting drunk and acting raunchy, and he managed to both kiss and feel her up in the center of the dance floor, he is not going to be happy when she goes out with her friends.

This is simply logical. No one likes to be embarrassed and betrayed. Now if he met her at the same club, yet she was moderate with drink, flirted coyly, and pushed his hands away when he tried to pull her close, he will be much less controlling about this.

Finally, the courage that a man possesses determines how he deals with competition. A cowardly man may be controlling even if he can logically trust his woman and normally cares about her feelings.

A heroic man has enough confidence in himself to express his desire to protect in a positive way. You can inspire healthy guarding by having a feminine appearance and manner and being friendly to others, including men.

If you have been working on your character and appearance, this will come naturally after some time. Let him see that other guys hit on you, including desirable guys. If a man is disrespectful and blatantly sexual, make it clear that this is out of line.

However, a man who is interested but respectful can provide an exciting challenge for your main squeeze. If you make it clear that this man is just a friend or colleague and perfectly harmless, you will look like the innocent, pursued party. Your dignity and sexual restraint proof this further.

You don't linger at men's apartments or make out with men you date in the streets, so on a rational level you cannot be expected to indulge in a dalliance. On an emotional level, the idea that you have the opportunity to do so flares up his competitive drive.

Thus, you provide an exciting game, that your beau knows he can win. Let him guard you like a princess, not a prisoner.

39- Give Him A Lasting Memory Of You

- Your marriage will be shaped by your habits. When you create a habit of consistently showing thoughtfulness to your spouse, he will remember it and treasure those memories.

These can be as simple as giving a nightly foot massage, hiding love notes around the house, sending text messages throughout the day just to say "I love you," or a million other things. Romance in relationship is about much more than big, one time events; it's about doing the little things with consistency and thoughtfulness. Those little things add up over time.

AND BEST OF ALL HOW TO ENJOY YOUR FEMININITY AND LET THE WORLD SEE IT

What is femininity? Femininity is a state appropriate to every woman and manifested in different shades and intensity. Some women are more aware of their femininity, others are not. The more we are aware of our femininity, the easier it is noticed by others.

Magnificent world of femininity often when we ask somebody how a very feminine woman looks like, a list of specific qualities that suggest femininity is offered. The set of all her feminine traits and qualities is her femininity.

Every woman has awakened in her being several wonderful qualities that give her a lot of charm and beauty. Some of us are more romantic, others more playful, others more courageous, more curious, more sensual, more passionate, more sympathetic, more maternal, more voluptuous, Many women are unhappy with themselves and while looking at other women they say how much they want to be like them.

And this is happening primarily for the reason that they are not aware of the qualities they have already, because they are not enjoying their own femininity. It is very important to be aware that each of us has a specific charm and that each of us if she wants to be more than she is right now and to amplify femininity, CAN do it.

If you were to take a trip into the world of femininity, what would you discover? We would find a lot of qualities, all fascinating and charming in its own way: naturalness, the power of love, dedication, mystery, sensuality, playfulness, purity, delicacy, compassion, sensitivity, passion, voluptuousness, wisdom, intuition, fascination, power to forgive, curiosity, sense of adventure, desire for knowledge, sense of humor, optimism, beauty, innocence, intensity, ability to appreciate beauty, ability to listen to others' needs and to help, tenderness, gentleness, patience, creativity, spontaneity, inner strength (often mysterious and overwhelming) power of sacrifice, intelligence, tenderness, romance and others.

Enjoy your femininity!If you have not recognized by now what a wonderful woman you are, you can do it now, it is enough to look closely at yourself. You can ask also your beloved ones to help you.

Make a list of your qualities and ask some of your close beings who are honest with you to tell what they appreciate at you. It may surprise you to find out that others see you as a beautiful woman and full of qualities. Look at this exercise as a journey into the world of your femininity and enjoy your beauty.

HOW TO GET A MAN'S ATTENTION USING YOUR FEMININITY

If you have trouble attracting men and getting a date, you may be unknowingly sending vibes that push men away. Men think differently than women, so you have to understand how the male psyche works in order to get his attention. Know what to do to grab his attention.

Play hard to get. The worst thing you can do is to smother a guy or appear desperate.

Men are attracted to the thrill of the chase, so if you're chasing after him, you're taking away the challenge. Keep it low-key and keep him on the edge of his seat. Maintain your composure. Your outward indifference may make him want you more.

Be mysterious. A huge part of attracting men is letting them figure you out. Don't talk his ear off about every detail of your life or your feelings. Carefully think about what you say and don't fill the conversation with idle gabbing.

Also, don't make yourself available all the time. Allow him to wonder where you are and what you're doing.

Display intelligence and depth. Don't say "like" and "um" in every sentence. Intelligence is sexy. A smart woman who knows what she wants and how to get it will attract men everywhere she goes. Displaying your intellect reveals that you have depth. This will attract men more effectively than coming across as dim.

Be fun, in ways that men think are fun. This rule of attraction seems simple enough, but so many girls get it wrong. Don't be too much of a stereotypical "girl." Be able to let your hair down and tell jokes, watch sports, play video games or poker with him and try to enjoy the things that he enjoys.

He's not interested in holding your purse while you shop. Nor does he care what happened on last week's episode of Days of Our Lives. Hang out at sports bars with him. He'll want you even more.

Take care of your appearance. A woman who takes care of herself will attract men easier than one who doesn't. Shower with nice-smelling bath products. Use a feminine scented deodorant. Brush your teeth well and always keep mints and gum on hand.

If you talk to a guy and your breath is less than fresh, he's not going to notice anything else about you. Keep your hair neat and clean and take pride in your looks. Use a perfume that smells sweet and sensual.

Dress to kill. Dress in clothes that make you feel sexy. You don't have to look like a tramp, just keep in mind the styles that are attractive to men. Wear feminine clothing that accentuates your figure and hugs your body just right. Use the colors red or pink to your advantage; remember, men are visual.

Flirt with body language. Lean in close to him when you talk. Touch his hand or shoulder during conversation. Smile and be genuinely interested in what he has to say. Turn your body toward him when you two are in close proximity. Don't make these flirting techniques over-exaggerated and noticeable, however. Let your natural flirtatiousness shine

OKAY; YOU'VE GOT HIM, NOW WHAT?

So here it is. After weeks of careful planning and a little scheming you've finally got the attention of that hot guy you've been drooling over for months. He's starting to talk to you a little more and giving you that eye contact that you've been wanting.

Things are on the right path but you also know that there are others vying for his attention too. So what do you do to get him to have eyes for only you? First of all, if you want to wrap this guy up, it's important to know your strengths and use them to your benefit.

If you're a great cook learn his favorite dish and make him a meal of his favorites that leave him coming back for more. If you're a talented writer, compose a cute, funny poem that'll leave him laughing. This will make him think of you every time he thinks about that poem.

These are just a couple of examples but the key is to know what you're good at and use it to your advantage to impress him. Also remember when you're trying to make a guy your one and only you need to dress the part.

This doesn't mean that you have to be in a miniskirt and stilettos every time you see him. That would be a little weird. Just don't forget to take the time to look nice everyday. Remember no one wants to hook up with a slob.

So take the time to put on a little makeup even if it's only blush and lip gloss and it's okay to have your hair in ponytail as long as it's well groomed. Want to really get a guys attention? Play up your common interests. Everyone knows most guys love sports. If you're an avid football fan, you've already scored huge points with most guys. Plus if the two of you like the same team that could put you over the top.

No matter what the common interests, make sure you use them to your advantage. Not only will this make you favorable in your guy's eyes, it will also give the two of you lots to talk about. Everyone knows it's a lot easier to be with someone when you have things in common with. Finally the main thing you need to remember when it comes to making the guy of your dreams your one and only is to be real.

``Most guys can smell a fake woman from miles away and there is nothing that's more of a turn off. Be yourself in all situations. This will not only help to cement a serious relationship but you'll also know that it's the real you that your guy's in love with and not some fake version of a woman you think your guy wants to be with.

Besides if you pretend to be someone else, the real you will always come to light at some point and time and you could stand to lose your guy if he finds out you've been lying to him all along. Save yourself some trouble and potential heartache by being real from the very beginning.

So now that you've got your guys attention and you want to go in and stake your claim on him you need to play it smart. The bottom line is if you got his attention in the first place then it's obvious his interest is piqued.

Just be yourself but at the top of your game. In other for you to be you at your very best, it may take a little time and patience but if he's smart (which I'm sure he is if you like him right) he'll come to his senses and snap you in a flash.

1ST CHAPTER OF MY BEST-SELLING BOOK: HOW TO BECOME A HIGH-QUALITY WOMAN

WHAT WOMEN NEED TO KNOW ABOUT LOVE, RELATIONSHIPS, AND MEN

What women need to know about love, relationships, and men. Wouldn't you love it if this little book had everything you ever needed to know about men in it? Well, I'm sorry it doesn't. But, it does have some great insights into the lives of men and what they are looking for in a woman to spend the rest of their lives with. This article speaks directly to all the single women out there... but it is a timely message for all of us all!

Have you ever had one of those weeks where it seems like messages or themes keep repeating themselves? It was definitely one of those weeks for me. The funny thing was what this theme was... I was like, really God; THIS is what you want me to write? I'm not kidding this theme and message showed up everywhere this week!

So, I know you are dying to know what it is I've heard all week. I want to warn you this will probably ruffle some feathers; but, I'm all about taking leaps of faith lately so here it is: "Men of worth do not marry vagina they marry virtue"

I've lost some of you already I can tell. But I'm serious stay with me here... just keep reading!

Men of Worth Marry Virtue

Let me first explain to you the context of the above stated quote. I was watching "Millionaire Matchmaker" on TV the other night and the resident therapist was giving one of their millionaire clients a few pointers about the difference between casual dating and finding love. What she told him was that if he wanted to be a man and find love he was going to have to do this differently. That's when she dropped the bomb, "Men of worth do not marry vagina. They marry virtue." It was like a light bulb went off in his head... I felt like cheering in my living room!

The definition of virtue is to have worth and to be of good quality or admirable. To all beautiful single women out there-so many of you are missing this! Somewhere along the way you've bought into the LIE that ANY man is better than NO man. Whether you are single or married, let's face it, some of you have given up the belief that you are worth fighting for or that you have anything admirable about you.

Some of you no longer feel like you are even worthy of a good man's love. That is a LIE! Some of you believe that they are no good men left so you settle for whoever is around. That is a LIE! Just because you've been treated like that in the past doesn't make it right or even the truth. Just because you haven't found a man of worth who will treat you like the virtuous women you are doesn't mean he isn't out there. Ladies, don't settle! Start to discover, and believe, your own worth. You were designed and made with a purpose and it wasn't to give up and settle.

A Love Story for the Ages

Ruth understood what it meant to wait for a man of worth to come into her life. The story of her life and her eventual marriage to a man of honor is in the book of Ruth in the Bible. Ruth was widowed at a young age in a time in history when it was not good to be without a husband or a son. In this time period all of society was structured around men and Ruth was left homeless, broke, and forced to rebuild her life alone.

Through faith, perseverance, one heck of a plan by her mother-in-law, and God's divine orchestration, Ruth found herself being wooed by the most eligible rich bachelor in town Boaz. She found a love that literally was a love story for the ages! If you haven't read the story yourself I urge you to do that and see how this single woman had the courage to go after what she really wanted.

Ruth and Boaz didn't have their story written for all to read and remember because they were mediocre. Nope, their relationship was special. It was one of mutual admiration, respect, love, and honor. They understood each others worth perfectly and treated one another so. Their story is given to each of us as an example. It is not a pie in the sky idea that is past its time. It is something that can happen to every one of us.

What About You?

Let's be honest. How many of you single women are waiting patiently for God to bring you your Boaz? How many of you are following a carefully thought out plan to weed out the bad guys from the good guys? How many of you are acting like you are someone of worth?

To all my married ladies... how many of us have our "Boaz" but have neglected to treat him like the man of honor that he is? Or, how many of us have let our "Boaz" forget our worth and get away with treating us like we are no longer worthy and desirable... and guys, how many of you have been OK with no longer trying?

I hope I got you thinking today... and maybe even challenged your thoughts and behaviors. I want to see you and your relationships succeed. If you need some help in this area I urge you to contact me and we can start working together to get you out of this cycle. I KNOW you are created for so much more and I want to see you start to believe that. Take a chance!

I want to share you with this awesome quote I saw floating around on a few statuses' on Facebook this week. It really sums up this topic nicely.

To all the women out there who are in a hurry to have a boyfriend or get married, a piece of biblical advice: Ruth patiently waited for her mate Boaz... While you are waiting for your Boaz, don't settle for any of his relatives... Broke-az, Po-az, Lyin-az, Drunk-az, Cheap-az, Lockedup-az, especially his third cousin Beatinyo-az. Wait on your Boaz and make sure he respects Yo-az."

WHAT MEN WANT

This is a question that must be especially troubling to women in the modern times. If we ask women directly they say that men confuse them and they don't understand what men are really looking for in a relationship. Times have indeed changed. Today women are asserting themselves in their newer role as sexually liberated career women in charge of their own destiny.

What men want: The struggle of the modern man
The change in the world with women asserting in every sphere of life has really affected the traditional view men had about their good old world. Modern man is struggling to find his place in the new world but surely he is also evolving to fit into the changing circumstances. As he is evolving his outlook of life, relationships and expectations from his partner are also changing. This might be confusing to women but it is necessary for women to understand, appreciate and deal with this new reality as much as men are dealing with the reality of a newly assertive, confident and independent women.

What Men Want: What are men seeking in a relationship?
Friends this is a complex question and it does not have a simple answer. But keeping in mind the ever-changing and evolving world around us, we can construct a structure of what men might be really seeking in a relationship.

To start with there should be a basic love-interest and attraction for a relationship to build on. Men in the core of their hearts desire a trustworthy, faithful partner who can eventually share his personal life. Men are seeking women with a balance of the feminine and masculine nature. He would like to have a woman in his life who can be gentle, caring, nurturing, compassionate and simultaneously assertive, independent and intelligent.

What men want: Assertive and supportive partner
He would be seeking a friend as well as a mother for his future children. Men would also like to relate to their women, talk to them and share a joke with them. Sense of humor and good communication skills are important. Men would be looking for women who are supportive and are not nagging. He would prefer his partner to be assertive but not abusive and angry.

What men want: Stimulating and exciting partner

He would like a partner who is stimulating and challenging and who puts her natural efforts in keeping the zing going on in the relationship. Commitment, closeness and long term bonding is also important for him. Exploring sex and novelty in sex "stimulate men" and women who can participate in these kinds of experiments in a relationship will be high in demand. He also wants a relationship that builds on camaraderie, respect for each other and sharing in a mutually beneficial way. Infact men really look for buddies in all relationships.

What Men Want: The physiology and psychological perspective and the various stages

Looking from the most physical and biological level we can say that men desire hot, sexy and a happening girl as portrayed by the mass media. He goes flat for the physical attributes and desires the super-women types. Here the urge is lust and sex in the primal form. But this does not stand for long and cannot stand for long as an isolated stage. From this primal stage there is a transition to the next stage where men would like to get into relationships which are little stable and which they can boast among their circle of influence and friends. Here men try to have the best girl in the town and the major criteria is show off and pride. This is a stage where men are trying to fit into the system and they are particularly concerned about what others think about his relationship and his girl. Further he expects that his relationship is based on truthfulness and mutual trust.

What men want: The stage of maturity

Next stage is of maturity. Here he is trying to find the real meaning of his life. At this stage the focus slowly shifts from him to her. Its about giving and sharing than receiving. This is a stage where relationships are experienced and encountered as a mix of the physical, mental, intellectual and spiritual realms. Here the focus is on giving selflessly, serve, share and sacrifice a bit. Its a stage where he thinks of forming long term bond. The focus is also to create a home based on creativity, intellect, ambition and a diehard positive spirit. The search is to find somebody who is on the same level with him and loves him for what who he really is rather than on the superficialities.

What men want: The interrelation of stages

All these stages can work out in an interrelated way and there is no fixed rule that one stage will move to the next stage. In fact, most of the times its a kind of mixed story but as age progresses we can assume that men move from the basal physical stage to the stage where they are searching for the true meaning of their lives. We can still try to put things in age perspective but it has to be clearly understood that most of the time things are just interchangeable and work in a complex interconnected way.

What Men Want: At the age of 20, 30 and 40
At the age of 20's its time to enjoy and be merry. Here men are trying to find a pretty woman and show off to the world. At 30's he expects little stability and sanity in his life and therefore he is expecting a partner with whom he can settle down and share his life. At 40's he is more sensitive and he is in the process of finding the true meaning of his life. Here there can be an awakening, reemphasising and rebuilding of the relationship all over again. Again let me emphasize on the fact that the numbers are not absolute and some men move faster to the next stage and some remain in one stage for their entire life and there are few who are a mix of everything.

What Men Want: Nine general traits that a Man expects from his girl in his life
1. He knows that he is not adequate and fully grown and he expects that she makes him want to grow and be a better man.

2. He wants to connect with the society and he expects that she gets along with friends and family.

3. He wants some peace in his life. The world is any way barking and shouting at him and therefore he wants a nagless partner.

4. A man is a man and he wants to feel confident as a man. He would love a girl who lets him be a man.

5. This one is the most important issue for him in the ever-changing world. He needs self-respect and a boost to his ego and therefore he expects a girl who can respect him for whatever he is without being judgemental.

6. Of course he is a great connoisseur of beauty and he expects that she is beautiful not only physically but in all other ways. It also means that she is intelligent, communicative, assertive, sexual and enterprising in bed.

7. Finally he expects a caring and loving girl who is a bit like his own mother.

What men want: Every Man is unique just like every woman
Knowing what men want is a really tough question and though I have tried to generalize it, it is better to approach your man as a unique piece of wonder as you yourself are. His needs and feelings may be as personal as is yours.

MY GIFT TO YOU CLICK THE LINK BELOW

https://nowthis.life/rac/

If this book helped you out in anyway, please help
me to help others by writing a review!

https://www.amazon.com/dp/B072FPBD22
Still, if you did not get anything new from this book or you were
not impacted in some way, I would still like to hear what you have
to say. Either way, I will know what am doing right or wrong and to
improve in the future. I wouldn't like to take your money and not
deliver. So please, take just 2 minutes to let me know what you think.

Everyone is searching for help on how to improve their lives for the
better and one thing they do look for are reviews. If this book has a lot
amazing reviews with great comments, they will buy the book and read
it and so the ripples effects of goodness spreads. But if it doesn't have
any great reviews and comments, they don't buy the book and read it.

I know this book can positively impact and help someone
and you can help that person by writing your
thoughts and takeaways from the book.

Additionally, I would like to read your review and hear how
this book has helped you in anyway at shape or form. My plan is to
print every single review and hang them on my home office wall
to read for inspiration and motivation throughout the day.

Your great review helps me personally to stay focused
and be able to validate all the hard work and lots of hours
invested in preparing this book for you.

https://www.amazon.com/dp/B072FPBD22

OTHER BOOKS BY BRYAN

www.ingramcontent.com/pod-product-compliance
Lightning Source LLC
Chambersburg PA
CBHW061352250726

48657CB00004B/1463